Community Health
Promotion Ideas
That Work

Community Health
Promotion Ideas
That Work

Community Health Promotion Ideas That Work

Second Edition

Marshall W. Kreuter

Nicole A. Lezin

Matthew W. Kreuter

Lawrence W. Green

JONES AND BARTLETT PUBLISHERS
Sudbury, Massachusetts
BOSTON   TORONTO   LONDON   SINGAPORE

World Headquarters
Jones and Bartlett Publishers
40 Tall Pine Drive
Sudbury, MA 01776
978-443-5000
info@jbpub.com
health.jbpub.com

Jones and Bartlett Publishers Canada
2406 Nikanna Road
Mississauga, ON L5C 2W6
CANADA

Jones and Bartlett Publishers International
Barb House, Barb Mews
London W6 7PA
UK

Production Credits
Acquisitions Editor: Kristin L. Ellis
Production Editor: Julie C. Bolduc
Editorial Assistant: Nicole Quinn
Associate Marketing Manager: Ed McKenna
Manufacturing Buyer: Therese Bräuer
Composition: Interactive Composition Corporation
Cover Design: Kristin E. Ohlin
Cover Photograph: © PhotoDisc
Printing and Binding: Malloy Lithographing, Inc.
Cover Printing: Malloy Lithographing, Inc.

The photos on pages 34, 64, and 80 are © PhotoDisc; the photos on pages 2, 120, and 148 are © Rubberball Productions.

Library of Congress Cataloging-in-Publication Data
Community health promotion ideas that work / Marshall W.
      Kreuter . . . [et al.].
         p. ; cm.
      Includes bibliographical references and index.
      ISBN 0-7637-0059-2 (alk. paper)
      1. Health promotion. 2. Community health services.
   I. Kreuter, Marshall W.
      [DNLM: 1. Community Health Services. 2. Health Promotion.
   WA 546.1 C7336 2003]
   RA427.8.C636 2003
   362.1'2—dc21

                                            2002156045

Printed in the United States of America
07   06   05   04   03   10   9   8   7   6   5   4   3   2   1

Contents

List of Figures   ix
List of Tables   xi
Preface   xiii
About the Authors   xix

Chapter 1   FINDING TRUE NORTH   1
Case Story: Why Do We Do What We Do?   1
   Case Analysis   5
Why Did Linda Undertake the Stress Management Project?   5
What Do Dr. Jameson's Actions Tell Us?   6
How Would You Assess the Approach Linda Took in Implementing
  Her Stress Management Project?   12
Realistically, Can a Staff Person Have Any Influence on Setting
  Program Priorities?   14
Summary   15
Endnotes   16

Chapter 2   USING DIVERSE SOURCES OF DATA   17
Case Story: Let's Take a "Comprehensive" Approach   17
   Prologue   17
   The Staff Meeting   18
   Thinking It Through   22
   Input from the Epidemiologist   25
   The First Draft   28
   The Draft   32
   Four Months Later   32
   Case Analysis   34
Types and Sources of Public Health Data   35
   Helpful Resources and Models   35
   Step 1: Prepare for the Community   37

Step 2: Collect Data for the Core Indicators   37
Step 3: Identify Locally Appropriate Indicators and Collect Data   37
Step 4: Organize and Analyze Data, Compile the Findings, and
    Disseminate the Information   37
Step 5: Establish a System to Monitor Indicators over Time   38
Step 6: Identify Challenges and Opportunities Related to Health
    Status   38
Finding Data   38
People: Experience, Perception, and Wisdom   41
A Cautionary Note   41
Using Local Data to Stimulate Local Action   42
    Local Use of Data   43
Summary   48
Endnotes   48

Chapter 3   PROMOTING PARTICIPATION
            FOR HEALTH   51
Case Story: The Court of Public Opinion   51
    Case Analysis   59
Participation   59
Why Is Participation Important?   60
Building Political and Public Support   67
Heightening Public Awareness: Strategic Thinking   73
Summary   75
Endnotes   76

Chapter 4   WHAT'S THE PLAN? IS IT WORKING?   79
Case Story: What Causes the Causes?   79
    Case Analysis   87
Assumptions   88
The Targets for Change   88
    Step 1: List Risk Factors   88
    Step 2: Differentiate Between Behavioral and
        Environmental Factors   89
    Step 3: Shorten the List   89
    Step 4: Determine Factor Importance   90
    Step 5: Determine Changeability   90
    Step 6: Create a Matrix   93
    Step 7: Set Objectives   95
Identifying the Causes   96
Generating Predisposing, Reinforcing, and Enabling Factors   98

G'Day: Australia's Diagnostic Approach   99
Evaluation: Staying on Course   104
    Finding Evaluation Evidence: An Example   109
Summary   112
Endnotes   113

Chapter 5   THEORY APPLIED   115
Case Story: The Old Horse   115
    Case Analysis   122
Theory: A Primer   123
    Is the Theory Relevant to My Problem?   125
    How Does the Theory Help Me Understand Targets
      for Change?   125
    How Does the Theory Help in the Selection or Development
      of an Intervention Method or Tactic?   125
Theory Summaries   126
    Health Belief Model   126
    Self-Efficacy   128
    Theory of Reasoned Action   131
    Diffusion of Innovations Theory   133
Community Capacity, Coalition-Building, and Social
  Capital Theories   138
Summary   143
Endnotes   144

Chapter 6   TACTICS   147
Case Story: Checkmate   147
    Case Analysis   152
Six Principles   152
    Principle 1: Use Objectives to Stay Focused   152
    Principle 2: Make Informed Decisions   153
    Principle 3: Don't Reinvent the Wheel   153
    Principle 4: There Is No Such Thing as a Free Lunch   153
    Principle 5: To Maximize Effectiveness, Strategically Combine
      Multiple Tactics to Influence Complex Problems   154
    Principle 6: Be Creative   154
Health Communication: Follow the Signposts   155
    Signpost 1: What Can Health Communication Do for You?   155
    Signpost 2: With Whom Are You Trying to Communicate?   156
    Signpost 3: What Does It Cost Your Audience to Hear
      Your Message?   157

Signpost 4: What Do You Want to Say?   158
Signpost 5: How Will the Message Get to Your Audience?   159
Media Advocacy: Addressing the "Manufacturers of Illness"   161
Enter Media Advocacy and Politics   162
Some Practical First Steps   163
If You Don't "Frame It" Correctly, They Aren't Likely
to Get It!   165
The Key: Anticipation   166
Scenario   166
Policy, Regulatory, and Environmental Actions   168
Policy and Regulatory Actions   168
Environmental Interventions   174
Reminders or "Prompts"   175
Be Ready to Use "Evidence"   176
Tailoring: Combining Technology with Theory   177
What Is Tailoring?   177
Tailoring Works!   178
How Are Tailored Materials Created?   179
Coordinate Multiple Tactics   184
Summary   186
Endnotes   186

Chapter 7   STEERING VERSUS ROWING   191

Case Story: Jameson   191
Case Analysis   197
Management and Organizations   198
Essential Services   199
Strategic Planning   199
Benchmarking   202
Private- and Public-Sector Enterprises   202
Budgeting   204
Management and Individuals   205
Information Flow   205
The Supervisory Relationship   206
Professional Development   207
Professional Identity   207
Summary   208
Endnotes   208

Index   209

List of Figures

Figure 1.1   Unaligned Team, *9*
Figure 1.2   Aligned Team, *10*
Figure 1.3   The Core Functions Applied, *11*
Figure 1.4   The Rise and Fall of *E. coli* Cases, *13*
Figure 2.1   Percent Colorectal Cancer Cases Diagnosed by Stage and Race, United States, 1992–1997, *28*
Figure 2.2   Five-Year Survival Rates by Stage at Diagnosis and Race, 1992–1997, *29*
Figure 2.3   Framework for Comprehensive Cancer Prevention and Control, *31*
Figure 2.4   North Carolina Child Health Report Card, *44*
Figure 2.5   Findings Related to "Experiencing" Discrimination, 2000, *47*
Figure 2.6   Findings Related to Discrimination as a "Problem," 2000, *47*
Figure 4.1   Accomplishments of the Our Kids Count Coalition, *83*
Figure 4.2   Factors That Influence Behavior, *84*
Figure 4.3   Rating Environmental Factors by Importance, *91*
Figure 4.4   Rating Environmental Factors by Changeability, *94*
Figure 4.5   Importance and Changeability Matrix, *95*
Figure 4.6   Predisposing, Reinforcing, and Enabling Factors, *96*
Figure 4.7   Factors That Influence Teen Drinking and Driving, *99*
Figure 4.8   Steps in Program Evaluation, *105*
Figure 6.1   Colonel Tim Gayle's Modification of the Reid et al. Table, *151*
Figure 6.2   Primary and Secondary Audiences for Oral Rehydration, *157*
Figure 6.3   Individual Profile Generated from a Theory-Based Survey, *183*
Figure 6.4   How Theory Guides the Tailoring Process, *184*

List of Tables

Table 2.1   Listed and Actual Causes of Death, United States, 1990, *23*

Table 2.2   Ten Most Common Diagnosed Cancers by Sex, 1999–2000, *26*

Table 2.3   Colon and Rectum Screening, Adults 50 and Older, United States, 1999, *27*

Table 2.4   Characteristics and Examples of a "Comprehensive Approach," *30*

Table 3.1   Communications Planning Matrix, *71*

Table 4.1   Preventing Pedestrian Injuries Among Five- to Nine-Year-Olds, *100*

Table 4.2   Environmental Factors: Volume and Speed of Traffic, Road Design, Roadside Obstacles, *102*

Table 4.3   Selected Baseline and Follow-up Indicators, *110*

Table 4.4   HLCC Quarterly Progress Log: Verified Changes in the Longview Community and Systems Environment Related to Tobacco-Use Prevention, *111*

Table 5.1   Diffusion of Innovations Theory, *135*

Table 6.1   Steps in Carrying Out the Key Tasks for Tailoring Health Promotional Materials, *180*

Table 7.1   Ten Strategic Planning Steps, *201*

Preface

What is a healthy squirrel? Not a picture of a squirrel, not . . . the sleeping squirrel, not even the aggregate of his normal blood pressure, serum calcium, total body zinc, normal digestion, fertility, and the like. Rather, the healthy squirrel is a busy-tailed fellow who looks and acts like a squirrel; who leaps though trees with great daring; who gathers, buries, and covers but later uncovers and recovers his acorns; who perches out on a limb. . . who chatters and plays and courts with mates, and rears his young in large improbable-looking homes at the tops of trees.[1]

For many people, the word *health* seems to be synonymous with the words *health care* or *diseases,* which in turn call to mind terms like *medicine, hospital, doctor,* and *nurse.* In creating the metaphor above, Leon Kass took a different tack and invited us to envision health in the context of living—in short, seeing what health looks like!

In preparing the second edition, as we did when writing the first edition of this book, we took Kass' advice and asked ourselves: What does community health promotion look like? This question prompted two others: (1) What do effective health promotion practitioners do? and (2) What ideas or thought processes seem to guide the decisions they make? Out of this process emerged a variety of actions and ideas, some of which were persistent. We call the persistent ones "ideas that work."

Great progress continues to be made in the science, theory, and application of health education and health promotion. Thanks to the combined good work of dedicated practitioners and researchers the world over, we now have a much more coherent picture of the theories, strategies, and tactics that lead to health improvement in communities.

In our collective travels over the years, we have had the great pleasure of observing, and often working with, health educators and public health advocates from Boston, Massachusetts, to Lagos, Nigeria; from Bethel,

---

[1]Kass LR. Medical care and the pursuit of health. In: Lindsay C, ed. *New Directions in Public Health Care,* 13rd ed. San Francisco: Institute for Contemporary Studies; 1980:16–17.

Alaska, to Abbeyville, South Carolina; from Perth, Australia, to Tianjin, China. It has been inspiring to see these health workers, often operating with meager resources, use their ingenuity to create the conditions that will put people in a better position to improve their health and quality of life.

Despite the good work, a gap unfortunately remains: the gap between what the evidence tells us works and what is actually being applied in the name of health education and health promotion. The motivation behind this book was our desire to contribute to the narrowing of that gap.

For those currently studying in preparation to apply health promotion principles and strategies in their work, and for those front-line practitioners in the field, we have tried to create a user-friendly book—one that tries to unpack the knowledge and experience gained by other researchers and practitioners. Throughout the book, we use the term "health promotion practitioner" to refer to both.

Community Health Promotion Ideas That Work is organized into seven chapters, each of which begins with a case story. Although fictional, the stories are based on real experiences and include nuances of the human condition that are too often excluded from the study of public health practice. The case stories offer readers a realistic frame of reference in which to consider the critical concepts, principles, and theories that guide effective health promotion practice.

Chapter 1: Finding True North

This chapter focuses on the core purposes of public health. The case story that launches this chapter poses a rhetorical question: "Why Do We Do What We Do?" It asks practitioners to examine the rationale used to determine how they spend their time and resources. The story chronicles the experiences of a young and enthusiastic health worker who plans and implements a health promotion activity that, on the surface, looks fine. When her efforts are juxtaposed with the core principles of public health and the realities of limited resources, we are all prompted to reexamine the assumptions we use, or don't use, when determining which health issues to address in our work.

Chapter 2: Using Diverse Sources of Data

The case story, "Let's Take a 'Comprehensive' Approach," describes how a health promotion practitioner contributes to the process of crafting the coming year's budget recommendation for the Health Promotion Branch of a state health department. Ultimately, the program must defend its decision before the legislative budget committee. The case story analysis and chapter content combine to highlight (1) the value of using a wide range of data and information to determine priorities, (2) methods that practitioners can employ to gather that information, and (3) ways that one might make the case for moving from categorical health initiatives to those that take a more comprehensive and robust approach.

Chapter 3: Promoting Participation for Health

"The Court of Public Opinion" describes how a temporarily disheartened local health officer is buoyed by a friend who is a local journalist. The story and analysis illustrate the importance of one of the core principles of health promotion: community involvement and participation. This chapter brings to light the political realities that accompany health promotion and disease prevention and offers practical strategies designed to help practitioners in their efforts to respectfully engage those disparate populations who are so often left out of the process. Specific methods for communicating with public and political leaders are also described.

Chapter 4: What's the Plan? Is It Working?

"What Causes the Causes?" shows how a determined community coalition, coached by a health promotion professor, tackled underage drinking and drug use in its community. By systematically identifying the factors contributing to this serious and complex problem, the coalition uncovers those most amenable to change. In the process, they also build a solid and realistic foundation for evaluation. Practical examples for implementing the processes planning and evaluation are provided.

Chapter 5: Theory Applied

Experience has taught us that the most effective health promotion programs are those that employ multiple methods, matched to the specific needs and unique characteristics of the target population. "The Old Horse" case story takes us to China and illustrates how selected theories, in combination with the understanding of cultural nuances, were applied to create an effective tobacco use prevention and control program. This chapter reviews seven theories: four that relate to the dynamics of behavior change and three that focus on selected factors critical to social and community change. A working knowledge of these core theories belongs in the repertoire of every health promotion practitioner.

Chapter 6: Tactics

The case story, "Checkmate," uses the analogy of chess to draw a distinction between the terms *strategies* and *tactics*. The *strategic* part of health promotion is akin to the process of program planning. The *tactical* part of health promotion emerges from the plan and is manifested by the selection and implementation of methods, in concert with one another, aimed at achieving the objective and goal of the program. This chapter provides practical, "how to" key tactics used by practitioners in the field, including health communication, media advocacy and policy tactics, and tailored communication.

Chapter 7: Steering Versus Rowing

In "Jameson," we return full circle to the setting and characters introduced in the first case story. The health officer seeks outside consultation to learn how his health department could spend less time "reacting" and more time "initiating." Managerial, organizational, and budgetary tenets, so critical to effective health promotion programs, often remain in the background of our thinking. In this chapter, those tenets are brought out of the shadows.

ON SOUND PROFESSIONAL GROUND

The content of *Community Health Promotion Ideas That Work* provides practical examples that complement the content and principles covered in the seven "areas of responsibilities" for the Certified Health Education Specialist (CHES). The seven areas of responsibilities, and the chapters that address them, are as follows:

1. Assess individual and community needs for health education (Chapters 1 and 4)
2. Plan effective health education programs (Chapters 2–4)
3. Implement health education programs (Chapters 2–6)
4. Evaluate the effectiveness of health education programs (Chapter 4)
5. Coordinate the provision of health education (Chapters 3 and 7)
6. Act as a resource person in health education (Chapters 4 and 7)
7. Communicate health education needs, concerns, and resources (Chapter 3)

To paraphrase the English statesman Lord Acton, ". . . ignorance and the love of ease are the natural enemies of progress . . ." Our intention has not been to create a "cookbook" that makes the process of health promotion "easy." While health promotion is certainly rewarding, it is not easy! Our goal has been to bring into sharper focus the central tasks of health promotion while not losing sight of the reason for doing them: health improvement. If readers make those connections, and do so with some ease, so much the better.

Acknowledgments

The content of this volume is the product of many researchers and practitioners who have shared their findings with us, either directly or through their published work. Recognizing that any attempt to list the "many" runs the risk of being incomplete; we take that risk nonetheless. Any omissions are unintended and should be attributed to our failing memories!

For their ideas and good work, we are grateful to David Altman, Zhang Baoyi, Bill Beery, Teresa Byrd, Ellen Capwell, Billie Corti, David Cotton, Donna Cross, Delisa Culpepper, Lori Dorfman, Michael Eriksen, Steve Fawcett, Jack Finch, Bill Foege, Stu Fors, Bob Gold, Bob Goodman, Sonja Greene, Yu Hai, Jim Herrington, Peter Howatt, Grade Imoh, Steve Jones, Bob Kingon, Lloyd Kolbe, Fred Kroger, Brick Lancaster, Richard Levinson, Dave Lohrmann, Bobby Milstein, Bob Moon, Chuck Nelson, Gary Nelson, Hod Ogden, Guy Parcel, Kathy Parker, Joe Patterson, Ken Powell, Pekka Puska, Amelie Ramirez, Glen Ray, Gayle Reiber, Barbara Rimer, Mark Rosenberg, Randy Schwartz, Vic Strecher, Marni Vliet, Larry Wallack, Nancy Watkins, Lynna Williams, Susan Zaro, and Dexiu Zhang.

We would also like to thank our friends and colleagues who agreed to be photographed among the composite characters depicted in the case stories in this second edition: Michele Chang, Charlie Chen, David Cotton, Sara Craig, Bob Kingon, Adam Koplan, Arthur Lezin, Linda Miller, Bobby Milstein, and Bob Pinner. Their good-natured cooperation helped us in our effort to convey visually the human side of the stories we tried to capture in writing. Troy Hall, who took many of the photographs, somehow found exactly the right expression for each portrait. Additional images were provided by the Health Communication Research Laboratory at the Saint Louis University School of Public Health.

This second edition would still be in the "thinking stages" were it not for the professional insights and gentle persistence of our editor, Kris Ellis of Jones and Bartlett Publishers.

Finally, we would be remiss if we failed to acknowledge the support and understanding given by those closest to us. Martha, Rusty, Char, and Judith—thank you.

Marshall W. Kreuter

Nicole A. Lezin

Matthew W. Kreuter

Lawrence W. Green

About the Authors

Marshall W. Kreuter, PhD MPH (Hon)   *Public Health Consultant*
Marshall Kreuter, retired from the Centers for Disease Control and Prevention in 2000, is a consultant to international, national, and state health agencies and private foundations. He has dedicated his career to enhancing the skills of practitioners and is the consummate teacher. Marsh cooks for friends and family, plays golf, and lives in Atlanta, Georgia, and Bigfork, Montana.

Nicole A. Lezin, MPPM   *President, Cole Communications, Aptos, California*
In the field of public health, Nicole Lezin is best known for her distinguished work in two areas: strategic planning/management and technical writing. In both arenas, she has helped public health professionals analyze and communicate critical issues in epidemiology, injury prevention, teen pregnancy prevention, oral health, community-based health promotion, and school health education. She spends her free time reading and accompanying her dog on walks to the beach and through the redwood forests of central California.

Matthew W. Kreuter, PhD, MPH   *Associate Professor of Community Health and Director of the Health Communication Research Laboratory, School of Public Health, St. Louis University*
Matt Kreuter is an expert in the design and evaluation of computer-tailored health communication programs addressing a wide range of health issues including, but not limited to, smoking cessation, dietary changes, physical activity, weight management, cancer screening, childhood immunization, occupational health, injury prevention, maternal and child health, and alcoholism recovery. In his family, Matt is the reigning Scrabble champion.

Lawrence W. Green, DrPH, MPH   *CDC Distinguished Fellow and Director, Office of Extramural Prevention Research, Public Health Practice Program Office, Centers for Disease Control and Prevention, Atlanta, Georgia*
Larry Green's record of scholarship is unparalleled in the fields of health education and health promotion. No one has done more to contribute to strengthening the scientific credibility of the field. The products of his ideas, and his research, have influenced public health policies and practices globally. He has homes in Atlanta and San Francisco and, outside of his academic endeavors, exercises regularly and works on his jump shot.

CHAPTER 1

Finding True North

Case Story
_____ **WHY DO WE DO WHAT WE DO?** _____

Linda Thomas had prepared for her first-ever presentation at the annual Georgia Public Health Association (GPHA) meeting just like every other task she undertook—with careful attention to details and great enthusiasm. That's the way the Thomas family did things.

In her presentation, Linda described how she had recruited a total of 51 volunteers for a stress reduction program from Clarkston High School and two businesses: the Oconee Garment Manufacturing Company—where most of the volunteers were women who did shift work on sewing machines—and Southern Electronics, a company that manufactured computer components. During the course of a two-month period, she had provided the volunteer participants with six one-hour sessions that included instruction in relaxation techniques, small-group discussions to examine the sources of stress, and instruction in low-impact physical activity.

The results from Linda's evaluation showed that after their participation in the stress management course, participants were much more likely than control group subjects to identify and manage stressful circumstances. Those who had participated in the course also reported higher job satisfaction than control subjects.

Linda was also elated when a friend invited her to leaf through the comments that some of the participants had written on the session evaluation: "Crisp and to the point." "Handled questions like a pro!" "Great enthusiasm."

At the barbecue social the evening after her presentation, Linda was introduced to Dr. Fran Martin, who was giving the keynote address the following day. Dr. Martin was a living legend of public health. Everyone knew who she was: former dean of the University of California School of Public Health at Berkeley and former senior White House advisor. Dr. Martin was most recognized for her courageous work in establishing primary health centers in Mississippi during the 1950s and 1960s. She was now in what she called "semi-retirement." In reality, she was as busy as ever: writing, consulting, and giving presentations such as the one she was delivering the next day.

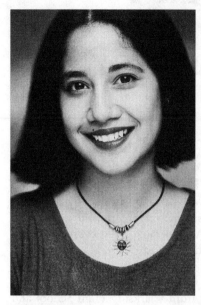

Linda Thomas

"It's really an honor to meet you, Dr. Martin." Linda's sincerity was genuine.

"Just Fran, everyone calls me Fran." She had smiling eyes and an easy manner.

"Incidentally, I attended your session today. Enthusiasm like yours is certainly contagious. Hang on to it!" Fran Martin was an engaging person who never seemed to be in a hurry; it was a pleasure to be in her company.

"Thank you. I noticed you in the back of the room toward the end of my presentation. I'm glad I didn't see you earlier, because I would have been even more nervous than I was."

Fran gestured toward a table. "Join me for dinner?"

Linda and Dr. Martin joined three others at a round table with a red-and-white checked paper tablecloth. The dinner conversation was lively and covered everything from gun control to the succulent barbecue. When someone jokingly asked Dr. Martin if she knew the health effects of eating barbecue, she paused, dramatically picked up a small juicy piece of barbecue with her fingers, and declared: "My motto is: All things in modera-

tion, but a taste of something a little sinful every now and then!" She promptly popped the morsel into her mouth to a chorus of cheers from her tablemates.

During the dinner conversation, Fran learned that Linda was formerly an elementary school teacher and had been working as a health educator for the Tri-County Health Department (TCHD) for just under two years. "How did you get interested in stress management?" Fran asked.

"About six months after I joined the Tri-County Health Department, I attended a wellness conference in Florida. I learned that high levels of stress are significant contributors to a variety of health problems and that relatively simple, low-cost exercises can alleviate stress."

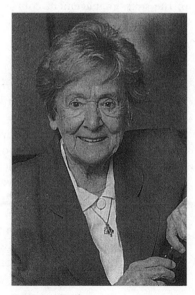

Dr. Fran Martin

Fran gave an understanding nod, and Linda continued. "While I was participating in the workshop, I felt the immediate benefits of relaxation and the breathing exercises." And then she lowered her voice to say, "Frankly, what the instructor was doing didn't seem all that complicated."

Fran chuckled. How refreshing it was to observe self-confidence!

Linda continued, "Anyway, after I got back from the wellness conference, I prepared a trip report and included a proposal to do a stress reduction demonstration program for personnel in selected schools and businesses within the Tri-County area."

"And your supervisor thought it was a good idea?" Fran probed.

"Actually, my regular health education supervisor had resigned to take another position and the county was in a hiring freeze, so my county health officer, Dr. Jameson, read the report. He told me that I could undertake the project as long as the program costs didn't have to come from the TCHD budget and if I did it without compromising my workload. Incidentally, Dr. Jameson will be here tomorrow to hear your presentation."

Fran could picture the position Linda's health officer had been in. In Linda, he had an employee with modest public health experience but great potential—a person with high energy and an intuitive knack for seeing and acting on opportunities to make things work. Fran could just imagine that Dr. Jameson wanted to nurture that potential and give her encouragement. Good personnel are hard to find, let alone keep!

The next day, Linda secured a seat in the front row at Dr. Martin's keynote address. The conference host took the podium and, after declaring that Dr. Martin needed no introduction, launched into a lengthy reading of her résumé. During the introduction, Fran caught Linda's eye and winked.

The person introducing Fran finally wound down, ". . . the title of her presentation is: 'Priorities for Whom?' Will you please welcome Dr. Fran Martin." Enthusiastic applause welcomed Dr. Martin. The applause stopped and the room was silent. Fran stood at the podium, looked down at her notes, and then slowly scanned the audience. In a clear, soft voice, she asked, "Why do we do what we do?"

The room remained silent. Then she asked rhetorically, "By what criteria are the human and economic resources of your organization or group assigned to actions designed to improve the public's health?" Everyone remained silent, awaiting the correct answer. Looking at the audience, she hunched her shoulders and partially extended her arms and asked, "Well?"

After another pause, she continued. "It's an interesting question, don't you think? What would serve as the basis for your response? Would it reflect some systematic assessment of the health needs of those you serve? Would it show that what you are doing is connected to what your organization stands for and is committed to? Would it reveal that the limited time and resources you have at hand are indeed being directed at those things that citizens perceive to be most important to their health?"

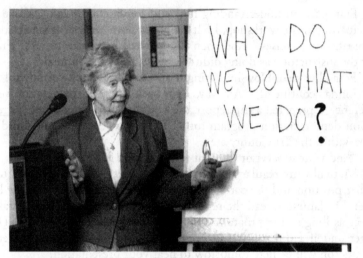

Dr. Fran Martin giving her lecture

Dr. Martin went on. "I find it useful to ask myself regularly, Why do I do what I do? If you remember nothing else in what I have to say this morning, please remember that simple question because I suspect that, like me, you will discover that your responses will lead you to insights you may not otherwise have considered."

The audience listened and thought. It was as if Dr. Martin were talking directly to each one of them. After jotting "Why do we do what we do?" in her notebook, Linda wondered to herself, Why did I undertake the stress management project? And she answered herself: I was informed that stress was an important issue. I found it to be an interesting approach, and those who experienced the program enjoyed it. And I have the interest and the ability to do it!

Dr. Martin was now into her presentation full swing. She showed slides of data comparing the leading causes of death, disease, and disability in Georgia with those of the rest of the nation. Then she showed a map of the southeastern portion of the United States and indicated that portions of South Carolina and Georgia are in what is called America's "stroke belt." She also pointed out that some of the states' highest rates of infant mortality and teen pregnancy are found in this same area.

She paused, then said, "You know, we have very good evidence that carefully planned health promotion programs can do a good deal to prevent these health problems and improve the quality of life not only of those who might otherwise have been needlessly victimized, but of their families as well." Knowing that she wasn't likely to get a response, Dr. Martin added, "Did you all know that?"

Linda fixed her gaze on the map—the Tri-County area was in the stroke belt. Pointing to the map, Dr. Martin continued, "At the risk of stating the obvious, I think we can do a much better job of putting into place programs that we know work. But to do that, we need to have better information, we need to digest and employ that information, and we need to be more focused."

Dr. Martin paused to take a sip of water and then added, "I can't remember who said it. Perhaps I did, long ago. Anyway, this quote seems quite appropriate here: 'The greatest obstacle to discovery is not ignorance, it's the assumption of knowledge.' I want to ask you to think seriously about what this means to your daily work."

As Dr. Martin made her closing remarks, Linda's thoughts darted back and forth between her stress management project and images of people suffering needless death and disability due to stroke and infant mortality. But my project was so well received, she thought.

Case Analysis

Most of us can identify with those who try to assemble a complicated device without first reading the instructions. We can go just so far before getting stuck, then spend a lot of our time and energy trying to get unstuck! The basic principles of public health offer us important guidance that can minimize the chances of getting stuck and ending up where we don't want to be.

Linda Thomas's experience in "Why Do We Do What We Do?" gives us a context to examine the practical relevance of some of the fundamental principles in public health—principles that are somewhat analogous to the instructions that came with that complicated device.

WHY DID LINDA UNDERTAKE THE STRESS MANAGEMENT PROJECT?

Linda's trip to the wellness conference in Florida was a positive personal experience. She learned that evidence links stress to a variety of health problems. Full of goodwill and good intentions, and armed with an interesting idea, she sought out an opportunity to apply and test her idea. She wanted to answer the following question: If people are taught stress management skills, will they report that the experience was beneficial and worth their while? Based on what we know from the story, the answer to her question was generally positive. Linda's experience is a good example of social learning theory in action. She had learned a new skill, gained confidence that she could use it, and demonstrated that she could apply it. Positive personal experiences are strong motivators; indeed, we tend to act on those things we do well, especially when our efforts are received with praise.

The story also forces us to acknowledge that while Linda was carrying out her stress management effort, another public health problem was apparently not being addressed. We know that the area served by the Tri-County Health Department had high rates of stroke, hypertension, infant mortality, and teen pregnancy. We heard Dr. Martin mention that the public health literature indicates that health promotion and disease prevention approaches have been effective in addressing the problems of stroke, hypertension, infant mortality, and teen pregnancy.

Here's the picture: We have a population where we can document priority health problems that affect a large number of people, and we have knowledge of effective interventions for these problems—but we have taken no apparent action. This raises a legitimate question: In the face of this information, was Linda's work on the stress management project the most appropriate use of her time and energy as a Tri-County Health Department health educator?

WHAT DO DR. JAMESON'S ACTIONS TELL US?

Linda Thomas is obviously a talented, energetic woman—all the more reason that her talents and energies should be focused on those activities most likely to have the greatest health benefit for the community served by the health department. But apparently no one, including her health officer, Dr. Jameson, raised the issue of the public health importance of what Linda was proposing to do. Why not?

Fran Martin had correctly assessed Dr. Jameson's position: he knew that Linda was a potentially outstanding employee and didn't want to discourage the initiative and enthusiasm she had demonstrated. What we don't know from the story is whether the Tri-County Health Department had a conceptual plan in place that would (1) help everyone see the direction in which the department was headed and (2) guide the distribution of its limited resources to the high-priority health problems and prevention strategies within its service area. As is the case for virtually all local health agencies, such a plan, in some form, probably did exist—but in all likelihood, it wasn't well communicated. Unfortunately, most local health agencies are understaffed and operate on shoestring budgets. When everyone's time and energy is spent on just keeping up, it takes a special effort to keep things from falling through the cracks.

Box 1.1, "Public Health in America," provides us with a general example of the key components of such a plan. It shows (1) the vision and mission of public health, (2) the six primary functions of public health, and (3) ten public health services deemed to be essential. The vision of healthy people in healthy communities reflects the condition that public health scientists and practitioners hope to achieve. The mission tells us how that vision will be achieved—through health promotion and disease, injury, and disability prevention. The six functions and the ten essential services indicate the actions or tasks that need to be carried out by public health workers. Note that the first two essential services listed involve assessing a community's health needs and investigating the determinants of health problems.

The public health perspective shown in Box 1.1 reveals a fundamental public health assumption: assessment of local needs is essential because

Box 1.1
PUBLIC HEALTH IN AMERICA

Vision

Healthy people in healthy communities

Mission

Promote physical and mental health and
prevent disease, injury, and disability

Public Health Functions

- Prevent epidemics and the spread of disease
- Protect against environmental hazards
- Prevent injuries
- Promote and encourage healthy behaviors and mental health
- Respond to disasters and assist communities in recovery
- Assure the quality and accessibility of health services

Essential Public Health Services

- Monitor health status to identify and solve community health problems
- Diagnose and investigate health problems and health hazards in the community
- Inform, educate, and empower people about health issues
- Mobilize community partnerships and action to solve health problems
- Develop policies and plans that support individual and community health efforts
- Enforce laws and regulations that protect health and ensure safety
- Link people to needed personal health services and assure the provision of health care when otherwise unavailable
- Assure a competent workforce
- Evaluate the effectiveness, accessibility, and quality of personal and population-based health services
- Research new insights and innovative solutions to health problems

Source: Baker EL, Melton RJ, Strange PV, et al. Health reform and the health of the public: forging community health partnerships. *JAMA.* 1994;272:1276–1282.

health problems and their causes vary from community to community. For example, the most prevalent health problems of children in rural Nigeria (malaria, diarrhea, lack of immunization) are not likely to be the same as those observed among children in Atlanta, Georgia (injuries, violence).

In the case of the Tri-County Health Department, it was Dr. Jameson's responsibility to make sure that all members of the TCHD, including Linda, understood what their organization's priorities were and why they were important.

Who wouldn't appreciate Dr. Jameson's support of Linda's display of initiative, considering the resignation of the area health education supervisor and the constraints on the Tri-County Health Department's budget? However, Dr. Jameson did Linda no favor by letting her move forward with so little counsel.

One of the primary duties of a supervisor is to help employees channel their good ideas and enthusiasm into directions that will help fulfill the vision and mission of the organization as a whole. Clearly, Dr. Jameson's decision to let Linda move forward with her idea without undertaking a critical review of how her proposed project stacked up against other possible program options is an important part of this story. Related to that point is a lesson for practitioners and managers alike. In delivering services to improve public health, *we cannot do it all.* With limited time and resources, the provision of services must be driven by rational criteria. Such criteria are reflected in the following simple questions:

- What are the documented needs of the people we serve?
- What are the perceived needs of the people we serve?
- What works?
- How does the proposed initiative fit in with the mission of our agency?
- What economic and human resources are available?

Most health promotion practitioners work in and for organizations like public health departments, volunteer agencies, schools, health philanthropies, and businesses. All of these entities have explicit purposes and goals that provide the guideposts for the directions they take.

For example, the Missouri Health Foundation (MHF) was created by the conversion from nonprofit to for-profit status by Blue Cross and Blue Shield of Missouri. The mission of the MHF is to improve the health of Missourians living in 85 Missouri counties and the city of St. Louis. In 2000, to help guide its grant-making strategy, the MHF asked the Missouri Department of Health to prepare a comprehensive analysis of health trends in its service area. In addition to providing detailed documentation of the leading threats to health in specific areas of the state, the final report recommended that the Foundation consider four guiding principles in its grant-making strategy:

- Are resources aimed at the highest priority and most serious threats to a population's health, including health disparities?
- Do resources support comprehensive interventions that engage multiple approaches and systems (e.g., clinical, public health, policy, behavioral, media)?
- Are resources invested in prevention efforts that can provide the most cost-effective solutions to reduce the burden of disease and the need for more costly long-term treatment?
- Are resources targeted toward interventions that have been shown to be effective?

This list prompts a rhetorical question: Had Dr. Jameson walked Linda through such a list, would the story have turned out differently? An organization's mission statement describes what the organization is trying to accomplish and how it intends to go about it. A mission statement that is shared by everyone in an organization is important precisely because the number of problems that the organization could potentially address far exceeds its capacity to address them all. Thus, if health workers understand and share a common vision and mission of their organization, they are more likely to be focused on priority issues and to be in sync with one another.

Boston Celtics basketball hall-of-famer Bill Russell has some sage advice to offer. He said that although the Celtics were a group of highly skilled specialists, their success depended ". . . both on individual excellence and how well we worked together."[1] Two figures graphically illustrate different scenarios.[2] In Figure 1.1, the arrows going in different directions reflect a group or team in which the members are out of alignment. Even though the individuals may work hard and have the best of intentions, their collective effort as a team will likely be incoherent and inefficient. In Figure 1.2, the alignment of the arrows suggests the kind of coherence and common purpose one would expect among members of an organization that share a common vision and mission.

Even when our role in an organization may be narrowly defined (e.g., adult health and chronic disease, school health, inspecting restaurants,

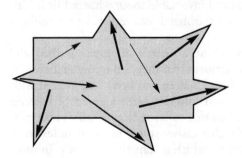

FIGURE 1.1 Unaligned Team

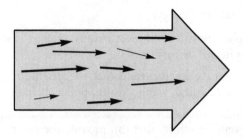

FIGURE 1.2 Aligned Team

immunizing children), vision and mission statements give us a framework for explaining how the specific tasks we perform fit into a larger picture—in other words, why we do what we do.

In 1988, the authors of *The Future of Public Health* described three core functions of public health: assessment, policy development, and assurance.[3] These functions, which are incorporated into the essential services listed in Box 1.1, are defined as follows:[4]

> ***Assessment*** is the regular collection, analysis, and sharing of information about health conditions, risks, and resources in a community. The assessment function is needed to identify trends in illness, injury, and death; the factors that may cause these events; available health resources and their application; unmet needs; and community perceptions about health issues.
>
> • *Short definition:* Figuring out what the important health problems are.
>
> ***Policy development*** is the process whereby public health agencies evaluate and determine health needs and the best ways to address them.
>
> • *Short definition:* Deciding what to do.
>
> ***Assurance*** refers to the actions taken to make sure that the needed health services and functions are available.
>
> • *Short definition:* Making it available and doing it right.

The core functions of public health reveal public health's broader framework and distinguish what is unique and invaluable about what public health workers do. To see how these ideas are translated into reality, let's consider a well-documented detective story.[5]

On January 12, 1993, officials at a Seattle hospital notified the Washington State Public Health Department that they had recorded increased visits for bloody diarrhea and that three children had been hospitalized with hemolytic uremic syndrome (HUS) and infection with a strain of bacteria known as *Escherichia coli* 0157:H7, hereafter referred to as *E. coli*. This strain of *E. coli* produces a powerful toxin that causes severe illness manifested as painful abdominal cramps and diarrhea, which is sometimes bloody. In most cases, *E. coli* infection results from consuming undercooked ground beef, raw milk, or contaminated water. The bacteria are present in the stool of infected persons and can be spread if proper hygienic practices are not followed. Among children and the elderly, *E. coli* infection can lead to the destruction of red blood cells, acute kidney failure, seizures, stroke, and even death.

On January 15, the health department initiated active surveillance throughout the greater Seattle area. By January 17, interviews with 37 patients revealed that 27 of them had eaten hamburgers from a particular fast-food chain, albeit at different outlets of the chain.

On January 18, Washington public health officials publicly announced the findings from a case-control study confirming that the cause of the outbreak was the result of the food preparation methods employed by a specific fast-food chain, wherein the meat processing had been improper and the hamburger patties had been undercooked. The announcement was accompanied with health education messages alerting food-service workers and the general public about the need to cook hamburger meat thoroughly.

Immediately after the January 18 announcement, the fast-food chain voluntarily removed the hamburger from its restaurants. In total, the outbreak resulted in 501 people becoming ill, three of whom died. Epidemiologists estimated that the action taken to remove 250,000 potentially contaminated hamburgers prevented at least 800 additional cases of illness. Thus 800 persons who would most certainly have gotten sick, some of whom may have died, didn't. Interestingly, we cannot know who those 800 people were. This tale provides a good example of why public health is often referred to as "the silent miracle." In a society where sensational media coverage predominates our information landscape, most of the media attention paid to the Seattle outbreak focused on the fast food, not the timely and effective response of public health workers.

As Figure 1.3 shows, the core functions of public health in Washington worked! Through a vigilant and active assessment, workers detected a serious

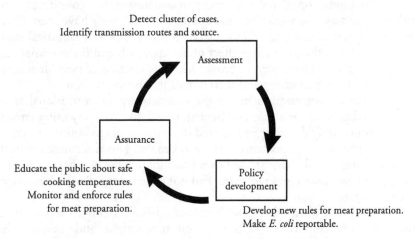

FIGURE 1.3   The Core Functions Applied

problem and tracked down its cause. Policy development required *E. coli* to be reportable and created systems to assure approved meat sources, proper cooking procedures, and timely public education.

Figure 1.4 shows the dramatic rise and fall of the *E. coli* outbreak. Behind these numbers and bars are real people, real families, and a real community. While some may cynically view the three core functions of assurance, assessment, and policy development as esoteric descriptors, we suspect that the people of Seattle see matters differently. It is understanding this broader picture of community health work that will help Linda Thomas keep her efforts focused in the future.

HOW WOULD YOU ASSESS THE APPROACH LINDA TOOK IN IMPLEMENTING HER STRESS MANAGEMENT PROJECT?

As you consider this question, keep in mind the second and fourth points under "Public Health Functions" in Box 1.1: protect against environmental hazards and promote and encourage healthy behaviors and mental health. Linda deserves high marks for her enthusiasm and her ability to work with multiple organizations to plan, implement, and evaluate a program. Based on the limited information given in the case story, it appears that Linda's approach was exclusively focused on promoting healthful behavior among the volunteers—equipping them with knowledge and skills to enable them to manage stress. However, we see no evidence that she took into account the conditions and environmental circumstances that might be giving rise to the stress the volunteers were trying to control. Is it possible that working conditions in the garment factory (e.g., temperature, noise, time on the shift, potential risk of injury) may have contributed to volunteer stress?

Had Linda considered the extent to which working conditions contribute to stress in the workplace, her approach would likely have been different. Behavioral science and educational theory, confirmed by empirical studies, suggests that the immediate effect of her approach and the sustainability of that effect would have been improved had Linda examined possible sources of stress in the environment and then moved to ameliorate them.

Unless an organization makes the commitment to institutionalize an educational program as a standard benefit, it will, like so many other efforts, be a one-time-only demonstration. Had the removal of environmental stressors been part of the approach Linda took, benefits gained through environmental changes could be sustained over time; those same benefits would also be enjoyed by newer employees who had not experienced the stress management program.

This is not to say that Linda's individual-skills approach was without merit—clearly, employees will benefit from new insights and competencies

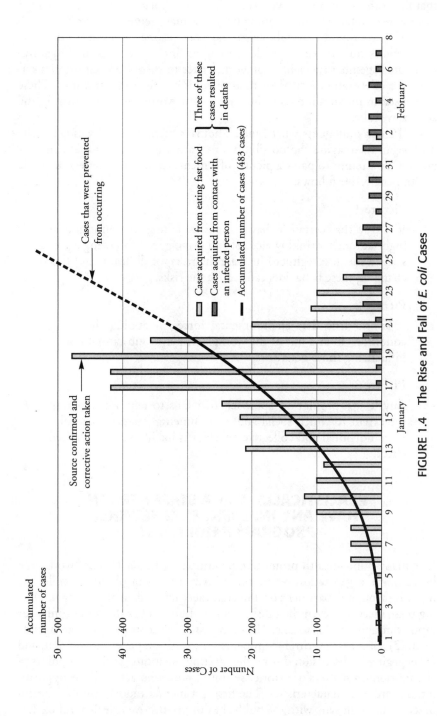

FIGURE 1.4 The Rise and Fall of *E. coli* Cases

that they can use outside as well as inside the workplace. What did Linda use as a frame of reference for planning her stress management effort?

We have found it useful to encourage practitioners to examine the basic assumptions they make when developing an intervention plan. Organizational management specialists sometimes refer to these basic assumptions as mental models[6] and describe them as pictures we carry in our minds. These subconscious pictures influence how we see the world and, consequently, the actions we take.

We can only guess what Linda Thomas's mental model was when she first began to imagine the possibility of creating a stress management program. Our attempt to paint a picture of a mental model that reflects a public health perspective follows:

Picture 1

It is true that certain behaviors (e.g., smoking, consumption of high-fat foods, drinking alcohol and driving, not following a prescribed medical regimen) increase the risks for ill health and that changing these behaviors can reduce the risks.

Picture 2

It is also true that environmental forces, including the living conditions in and out of the workplace, play a substantial role in influencing those behaviors.

Picture 3

Any health promotion approach that fails to take into account the extent to which social and environmental factors may influence individual and collective behavior is likely to have a limited effect.

REALISTICALLY, CAN A STAFF PERSON HAVE ANY INFLUENCE ON SETTING PROGRAM PRIORITIES?

Like many public health promotion practitioners, Linda Thomas works in a bureaucratic organization where the primary means of obtaining collective input is through department or unit staff meetings and email messages. During these meetings, even the most junior staff person has the opportunity for input through several means: (1) submitting or recommending an agenda item, (2) submitting written comments on a position paper or proposal, and (3) engaging in discussion during the meeting, including asking for points of clarification on matters of priority setting. Those who act on these opportunities share two characteristics. The first is a mental model of public health practice that is in sync with the public health perspective revealed in Box 1.1.

The second is simple: a willingness to raise questions and to learn. Although the latter characteristic came naturally for Linda, she apparently came up short on the former. Practitioners who view themselves as participants and are aware of and respect the principles of public health will have no problem.

SUMMARY

Dr. Martin's opening rhetorical question is meant to give us all a nudge; it challenges us to articulate the assumptions behind our decisions and to make sure that they are sound and defensible. It is a question that all practitioners, not just newcomers like Linda Thomas, need to call to mind more often. Our failure to ask "Why do I do what I do?" is not surprising when you think about it. The demands of our daily work routine tend to push our ultimate goals and purposes into the background. It is in such circumstances that we find ourselves driven by the question of "How should we do this?" rather than "Why is this important?"

This process of inquiry is a continuous one; we don't suddenly arrive at an answer that maps out our daily activities for the next five years. Assumptions and the decisions that flow from them can and should be adapted to changing conditions.

What does this have to do with identifying sources of information and obtaining data? Assumptions should be based on the best information available. As we will see in Chapter 2, this information will come from a variety of sources, including social and economic indicators, the perceptions and view of community residents, and epidemiological data. As public health practitioners, we have a responsibility to be familiar with the broad picture of health status in our communities—a picture that Linda Thomas had not yet painted for herself. (If she had, she would have known of and thought about the stroke belt and its implications for her proposed use of resources.) We also have an obligation to obtain relevant data if they are not immediately available, and to apply them skillfully to the problem we are trying to solve.

A wide gulf often exists between perceived and real threats to community health. Would you guess that more women die each year from breast cancer or lung cancer? Many people would guess that more lives are lost to breast cancer, but they would be wrong. A person who has lost a family member to breast cancer is naturally convinced that breast cancer prevention and treatment efforts should be a high priority; however, a family affected by diabetes may feel equally strongly about devoting resources to the disease that has ravaged its members. Is one issue more important than the other? Not necessarily. But we often have to choose among equally compelling needs. Data on the relative impact of risk factors and diseases can be one tool in justifying the use of public resources to address community health problems. It is also important to understand the perspectives and priorities of the people living in the community. Armed with sound and relevant information and data, health promotion practitioners will be able to set priorities, allocate scarce resources, and, last but certainly not least, determine the extent to which their efforts result in health improvement. Archie Graham faces these issues in the next chapter.

ENDNOTES

1. Russell W, Branch T. *Second Wind: Memoirs of an Opinionated Man.* New York: Random House; 1979.
2. These diagrams were taken from Senge P. *The Fifth Discipline.* New York: Doubleday; 1990:234–235.
3. *The Future of Public Health.* Washington, DC: National Academy Press; 1988.
4. These definitions of the "core functions" are taken from *Public Health Improvement Plan: A Progress Report,* Washington State Department of Health, March 1994. We found this document to be an excellent and practical blueprint for strengthening the capacity for public health. For a copy, contact: Office of the Secretary, 1112 SE Quince Street, P.O. Box 47890, Olympia, Washington 98504-7890.
5. Technical information on this example of an *E. coli* infection outbreak was taken from a paper written by Dr. Beth Bell and her colleagues: Bell B, Goldoft M, Griffin P, et al. A multistate outbreak of *E. coli* 0157:H7-associated bloody diarrhea and hemolytic uremic syndrome from hamburgers. *JAMA.* 1994; 272:1349–1353.
6. Again, we refer you to Peter Senge's *The Fifth Discipline.* In Chapter 10, he provides a detailed description of mental models. Time spent thinking about your mental model for health promotion planning, implementation, and evaluation is time well spent.

CHAPTER 2

Using Diverse Sources of Data

Case Story
___ LET'S TAKE A "COMPREHENSIVE" APPROACH ___

Prologue

Governmental health agencies at the national, regional (state and provincial), and local levels have much in common. Although their organizational configurations and economic bases may vary, all share a common goal: health promotion and disease prevention. They also share a common problem: finite resources available to address health problems that often seem infinite. Those responsible for approving budgets and allocating public resources do so based on priorities that have been established after careful consideration and debate.

Within state health departments, the process begins when programs try to craft a proposal strong enough to survive the scrutiny and politics of the budget process. That starting point provides the context for the case story that follows.

Before reviewing the case story, however, let's walk through a general review of how government checks and balances influence the allocation of public health resources.[1]

For most state public health agencies, the largest portion of their budget for health promotion and disease prevention will come from categorical grants they receive from the federal government.[2] In many instances, that portion will be as high as 90 percent. The remaining portions will come from their state budget appropriation and, in some instances, from grants made by philanthropies. Although smaller, the state budget appropriation is important because it allows the state to address priorities not covered by federal grants or to pursue further those health priorities that can be only partially met by existing federal support.

Each year, state governments are required to pass into law a state budget. Usually a budget has two elements: (1) the costs for maintaining existing programs and services and (2) the proposed costs for new initiatives. In this process, the executive branch of government (the governor) generates a budget based on needs reported by the directors of state government departments (e.g., education, transportation, health and human services). The governor's budget is then sent as a proposed bill to a body of the state legislature, usually a budget appropriations committee. Based on budget hearings and other discussions and debate, the committee modifies the budget and proposes legislative approval of the amended bill. More debate and compromise follow, until the bill finally passes through the legislative process and is returned to the governor to sign into law.

Budget proposals lacking credible and compelling evidence have little chance of surviving the budget process. At the same time, proposals grounded in credible and compelling evidence, absent political support and will, often finish as runners-up.

The Staff Meeting

Archie Graham grabbed a bagel from the passing tray as he listened to a review of the minutes from last month's staff meeting. Staff meetings of the state health department's Health Promotion and Chronic Disease Prevention (HPCDP) Branch in no way resembled the stereotypical picture of a gathering of bureaucrats. They were focused, lively, informative encounters that relied on staff input and participation.

The updates kept everyone informed. Elaine Elkins had reported on the success and statewide media coverage of a series of sting operations aimed at identifying businesses that sold tobacco products to underage youth. Elaine was also on the search committee to find a replacement for Janet Roy, coordinator of the breast and cervical cancer program, who had left to attend graduate school.

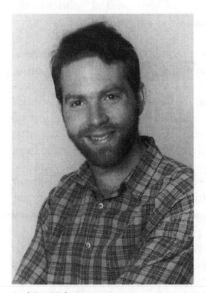

Archie Graham

"Interviews are scheduled in two weeks, and we hope to have the position filled a month or so after that." Elaine was acting in Janet's role and was eager to turn it over to the newcomer.

Bruce Willett, the coordinator for the Behavioral Risk Factor Survey, gave an update on CDC's plan to oversample large population areas to give states more local-level risk factor data. Margie O'Bannon provided an update on House Bill 462, a measure to create a statewide osteoporosis prevention program to be housed in the HPCDP Branch. At the conclusion of her report, Marge asked the group to give a warm welcome to Bill Minor, who just returned from his annual weekend ski trip to Colorado. Bill, wearing a cast from his left knee down, smiled, said nothing, and bowed as the staff gave him polite applause.

Three months earlier, Archie had joined the branch as a Public Health Prevention Specialist (PHPS) from the Centers for Disease Control and Prevention (CDC). PHPSs go through a three-year postgraduate, on-the-job training program; they are typically assigned to positions that offer opportunities to apply science-based principles and models in the design, implementation, and evaluation of prevention programs. In their first year, PHPSs have assignments in two different program areas within the CDC, with each assignment lasting about six months. The second and third years are served in a state or local health agency. Even though Archie had been on board for only a short time, he felt like part of the team. He felt fortunate to have this assignment — it was a good group.

Much of the credit for that belonged to the person who led the team. Judith Westphal was the chief for the HPCDP Branch of the state health department. An experienced public health worker, she had originally been trained as a public health nurse and later had completed an MPH in public health education. She was recognized by her supervisor, Dr. Joseph Jackson, Director of the State Health Department, and by the workers in her branch as a consummate supervisor. Dr. Westphal had high expectations of her staff, but always provided them with whatever support and guidance were necessary to ensure that their tasks could be successfully completed. She involved the staff in decision making, delegated important projects to them, and gave them responsibility and autonomy to complete the work. When giving assignments, she provided clear instructions and set reasonable deadlines.

Dr. Westphal had led the HPCDP Branch since its inception five years ago, when it was established as a new organizational component in the state health department during a reorganization. HPCDP was formed by combining the health education unit, which was part of the director's office, with three other programs: smoking and tobacco, cardiovascular health, and cancer control.

The main topic for today's branch meeting was the HPCDP budget proposal for the next fiscal year. "It's that time of the year," Dr. Westphal began, "time to begin preparing for next year's budget appropriation from the state. Given the rather bleak

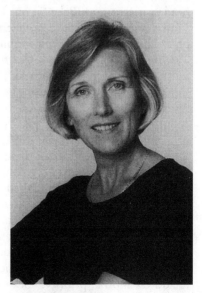

Dr. Judith Westphal

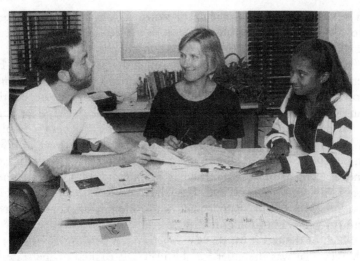

The HPCDP staff meeting

economic picture, the pool of resources for new initiatives will be much smaller than it has been in past years. Chances are, there'll be only enough money for one new project, if that, for our program."

She continued, "I spoke with Dr. Jackson yesterday and he assured me that all reasonable proposals from the branches would be considered for inclusion in the department's final budget. Recall that I asked all of you, during your last round of site visits to the local health districts, to poll them on the priority issues we're facing." Judith turned, placed a transparency on the overhead projector, and clicked it on. The slide showed a list of 15 priority topics. "You can see that the process generated a rather diverse list, but this one stood out." The shadow of her finger pointed to a category labeled *cancer prevention and control (lower-income, disparities).*

"Ten of our 12 local health districts[3] cited this as a priority. When I showed the list to Dr. Jackson, he seemed pleased because the governor and several legislators had expressed the view to him that 'more needed to be done about cancer'." Judith shrugged her shoulders and gestured by turning her palms up, "So, what do you think?"

Elaine Elkins spoke up first: "Four of the five districts I visited ranked breast and cervical cancer high and it kind of surprised me."

"Why is that?" Judith asked.

Elaine thought for a moment and then said, "I guess it's because, like all states, we have one of the CDC breast and cervical cancer grants and people at the local level appear to be pleased with the way it is going."

Judith offered a rhetorical question: "So if we are already getting support for a program that seems to be progressing well, why not go for resources to address another priority?" Several people gently nodded in assent.

Archie Graham wondered out loud, "I don't know—two weeks ago I did my first site visit to the Tri-County health district and they indicated that even though the breast cancer screening campaign was raising people's awareness and more women were getting mammograms, a sizable number of eligible women still weren't being reached. I don't have my notes here, but I think Tri-County staff said something about being surprised that more providers were not participating in the program."

Judith turned to Bill Minor. "Bill, the summary of your district report indicated that they were concerned about other cancers. Can you say more about that?"

"Sure. That was in the metro area, District 6. The health director, Ann Moore, expressed concern that the district incidence rate of colorectal cancer for males, during the period of 1998–2000 as I recall, was 15 percent higher than the overall state rate and 20 percent higher than the overall U.S. rate. During that same period, the early detection of breast cancer had improved at a rate consistent with the improvements noted in the rest of the state. However, no resources had been earmarked for colorectal screening and prevention."

After 10 minutes of further discussion, the group came to agreement that it made sense to move forward with a budget proposal that took a comprehensive approach to cancer prevention. The most compelling points were that it (1) would build on the foundation and momentum created by the breast and cervical cancer program, (2) appears to be a priority for the governor and several other political leaders, (3) emerged as a top priority for workers at the local level, and (4) should highlight the opportunity to address the issue of health disparities, which was a statewide priority.

After the meeting, Judith asked Archie to join her in her office. She explained that the task of crafting a first draft proposal would normally have gone to Janet Roy. With Janet's untimely departure, Dr. Westphal wondered, would Archie be willing to take it on? He was pleased to be considered and made it clear that he was happy to do so.

The two spent 15 minutes discussing various aspects of what Archie would be doing. Judith summed up the job: "Your task is pretty straightforward: create a first draft of the rationale we will use in the budget proposal. We'll add in the budget numbers later." She handed Archie a list of names, one of which, Gary Lee, was circled. "Gary is the state chronic disease epidemiologist. I suggest you waste no time getting to know him. In fact, I'll give Gary a call and advise him that you will contact him."

Judith scanned the calendar on her computer screen. "Budget proposals are due in the governor's office in about two and a half months. Let's see, today is the 7th, so why don't we plan to meet here in my office on the 30th at 10 a.m. to see where we are. Will that give you enough time to come up with a first draft?"

"I think I can do it." Archie had three weeks.

Thinking It Through

Archie went straight to his office. His "office" was, in fact, a cubicle walled off by dividers. A 3′ × 5′ white marking board was secured to one of the walls—he used that a lot. Archie also had a desk, computer, small bookshelf, and putty-colored filing cabinet, all of which were "previously owned."

Archie sat at his desk and began studying the few notes he had taken in hopes of finding a starting place. He thought for a while and then turned to his white board. In the middle, he drew a small box and in it inserted the words "breast and cervical cancer." He then pulled open one of the drawers in the filing cabinet and found a copy of *Cancer Facts and Figures* he had gotten from the local American Cancer Society affiliate. A table titled "Estimated Cancer Cases and Deaths by Gender, United States, 2002," listed 55 categories or "sites" of cancer. Archie jotted down about 15 of those cancer categories on the white board, encircling the box labeled "breast and cervical cancer."

In his notes Archie has underlined two words several times: *comprehensive* and *prevention*. *Comprehensive*—what did it mean in this context? Looking back at the board, he thought to himself, "By definition, the breast and cervical cancer program is categorical. But some of the local health districts mentioned colorectal cancer and oral cancer [indirectly identified by the reference to smokeless tobacco]. Does *comprehensive* mean adding other cancers to the programmatic mix?"

As Archie studied the board, he wondered what those various cancers might have in common. *Prevention*—he thumbed through *Cancer Facts and Figures* and found the heading "Can Cancer Be Prevented?" He read on:

> All cancers caused by cigarette smoking and heavy use of alcohol can be prevented . . . about one-third of the cancer deaths predicted for the coming year will be related to nutrition, physical inactivity, obesity, and other lifestyle factors . . . certain cancers are related to infectious exposures, e.g., hepatitis B virus (HBV), human papillomavirus (HPV), and others which could be prevented by behavioral changes, vaccines, or antibiotics . . . skin cancer can be prevented by protection from the sun's rays.[4]

The clear message was that several factors are known to contribute to more than one type of cancer. That made Archie recall a classic paper by Michael McGinnis and William Foege[5] in which the authors juxtaposed the 10 leading causes of death with what they termed the "actual" leading causes of death (Table 2.1).

As he reexamined the nine "actual" causes for mortality, Archie noted that six were directly related to several types of cancer: tobacco consumption, diet and activity patterns, alcohol, sexual behavior, certain infections, and toxic agents. Archie was beginning to get some insight into what *comprehensive*

TABLE 2.1   Listed and Actual Causes of Death, United States, 1990

Leading Causes of Death	Number	Actual Causes of Death	Number
Heart disease	720,058	Tobacco	400,000
Cancer	505,322	Diet/activity patterns	300,000
Cerebrovascular disease	144,088	Alcohol	100,000
Unintentional injuries	91,983	Certain infections	90,000
Chronic lung disease	86,679	Toxic agents	60,000
Pneumonia and influenza	79,513	Firearms	35,000
Diabetes	47,664	Sexual behavior	30,000
Suicide	30,906	Motor vehicles	25,000
Chronic liver disease	28,815	Drug use	20,000
HIV infection	25,188		
Total	1,757,216	Total	1,060,000

Sources: For leading causes of death, National Center for Health Statistics; for actual causes of death, McGinnis and Foege, 1993.

might mean. He picked up the phone and called Gary Lee. Gary had gotten a heads-up from Judith and told Archie that he had some time available between 2:00 and 3:00 the next afternoon. The two men agreed to meet in Archie's cubicle.

The next morning, Archie was able to schedule a meeting with Judith. He believed that the proposal would have added strength and credibility if it reflected the realities being faced by the local health districts. To get that perspective, he proposed conducting some brief follow-up telephone interviews with a sample of representatives from the health districts in the state and outlined his thoughts on how that process might be carried out. Judith thought the interviews were a good idea and, after discussing the details, they agreed on the following steps:

- Try to get input from 50 percent of the district health officers (or their designees)
- Stratify the sample of districts by geography and population density
- As HPCDP staff members were assigned to coordinate state-level activities with specific districts, use them as a point of contact for the telephone interviews
- Develop a structured interview guide
- Orient staff members to the interview guide to enhance the consistency of administering the survey and recording the responses
- Analyze the responses and incorporate them into the proposal

Judith sent an e-mail informing the staff members that the telephone interview strategy was a priority. She asked them to be prepared to set up their interviews up as soon as it was convenient for the health directors.

In his afternoon meeting with Gary, Archie began by describing the aims of the proposal and the interview process. He also shared his preliminary thinking about what the term *comprehensive* meant in the context of a cancer proposal. Gary suggested to Archie that he consider including an interview question like the following: If the state provided resources to support a comprehensive cancer prevention program, what would *comprehensive* mean to you?

When asked if he could help identify some data sources relevant to the proposal, Gary thought for a moment and then said, "It seems to me that local data would be the best. On that matter, I've got good news and not-so-good news!"

"The good?"

"For the past two years, the state has been working with the local districts to develop better 'small area' data, especially for chronic diseases, injuries, and related risk factors. And our state, like almost all states in the United States, has a cancer registry that enables us to report cancer data by age, sex, and race/ethnicity, to the county level. The registry includes accurate data about cancer incidence, stage at diagnosis, first course of treatment, and deaths."

"And the not-so-good?"

"It's mostly about time and readiness. At this point, only about one-half of the health districts in our state are systematically assembling and using local-level data. The data from the cancer registry will someday be a great resource, but we are just now beginning to get the capacity in place to utilize the data effectively."

"Why is that?" Archie asked.

"Because some of our counties are so small, they yield comparatively small numbers of cases. With such small numbers, you get a wide fluctuation of rates from one time period to the next and, even if you see differences, they are rarely statistically significant. This requires us to do two things: (1) use multiyear time periods and (2) find efficient ways to aggregate data from multiple counties into *district* data."

Sensing that his comments were less than inspirational, Gary added, "I know you've got a tight timeline and I think I have a feel for where you're trying to go. Let me see what I can come up with, and I'll get back with you." It was Thursday, and the pair agreed to meet on the following Monday in Gary's office because Gary had to leave for a meeting at CDC in Atlanta on Tuesday.

Archie developed a first draft of the interview guide consisting of five questions, including the question Gary had suggested. The questions were designed to prompt feedback from the districts on their prevention priorities, assets and strengths in carrying out prevention programs, major barriers, and priority resource needs. Archie gave the draft to HPCDP staff members and then revised it based on their comments and suggestions. Bill Minor and Marge O'Bannon did a mock runthrough—it took 22 minutes.

Input from the Epidemiologist

Gary was well prepared for his next meeting with Archie. He had gone through the most recent report of cancer incidence and mortality published by the state cancer registry to capture data that he thought Archie might be able to use in making the case for a comprehensive approach in his proposal.

"Here is a table [Table 2.2] of the 10 most common diagnosed cancers in our state by sex. Keep in mind that we have a population of just over 4 million. As you know, seven of those cancers (colon and rectum, lung, melanoma, breast, invasive cervix, prostate, and bladder) are either preventable or detectable at an early *and more survivable* stage of disease. And, if you go to the 'Both Sexes' column and add up the percentages for each of those seven, you'll see that the total comes to just about 65 percent."

"You think there's a message there?"

Archie nodded. "A very strong one."

Recalling Archie's early comments that some of the districts had reported that they needed to address different cancer problems, Gary wanted to see whether there were any geographic differences in trends in the state. "I looked for comparisons among the larger counties using age-adjusted incidence and mortality rates per 100,000 for the years 1998–1999 and 2000–2001. To start with, I looked only at trends in breast, prostate, and colorectal cancers."

Gary had created two sets of summary sheets and now handed one to Archie. The county mortality and incidence rates for breast cancer in counties were generally consistent with the overall state trend. And the trend was positive in that the percentage of cases detected in early stages (in situ and localized) had changed from 70 percent in 1998–1999 to 76 percent in 2000–2001. This 6 percent improvement was generally attributed to the benefits of early detection. However, Gary also found that five counties had early detection rates of 65 percent or less during both time periods.

The trend for prostate cancer in the state was also generally positive. The early detection of prostate cancer increased from 80 percent in 1998–1999 to 84 percent in 2000–2001. However, as was the case with the national trend, the incidence rate in blacks[6] in 2000–2001 was 40 percent higher than the rate for non-Hispanic whites and the incidence rate for Hispanics was 17 percent lower than the rate for non-Hispanic whites. As with breast cancer, Gary was able to identify seven counties where the early detection rates for 2000–2001 were 74 percent or less compared with the state rate of 84 percent.

Gary's analysis for colon and rectal cancer revealed a different picture with respect to the stage at which colorectal cancer cases were diagnosed. For example, the statewide rates for the early detection (in situ and localized) were

TABLE 2.2 Ten Most Common Diagnosed Cancers, by Sex, 1999–2000

Rank	Male Site	N	%	Female Site	N	%	Both Sexes Site	N	%
1	Prostate	10,453	29.0	Breast	13,686	36.6	Breast	13,750	18.7
2	Lung and bronchus	4520	12.6	Colon and rectum	3808	10.2	Prostate	10,453	14.2
3	Colon and rectum	3999	11.1	Lung and bronchus	3446	9.2	Lung and bronchus	7966	10.9
4	Melanoma	2468	6.9	Melanoma	2093	5.6	Colon and rectum	7807	10.6
5	Bladder	2303	6.4	Corpus uteri and uterus, NOS	1909	5.1	Melanoma	4561	6.2
6	Non-Hodgkin's lymphoma	1503	4.2	Ovary	1421	3.8	Bladder	3084	4.2
7	Leukemias	1032	2.9	Non-Hodgkin's lymphoma	1285	3.4	Non-Hodgkin's lymphoma	2788	3.8
8	Kidney	1029	2.9	Other and ill-defined	928	2.5	Corpus uteri and uterus, NOS	1909	2.6
9	Other and ill-defined	825	2.3	Thyroid	857	2.3	Leukemias	1782	2.4
10	Pancreas	784	2.2	Invasive cervix	846	2.3	Other and ill-defined	1753	2.4
	All cancers	36,009	100.0	All cancers	37,382	100.0	All cancers	73,391	100.0

Notes: The table excludes cervix in situ, benign brain tumors, and basal and squamous cell carcinomas of the skin.
Data presented in this table are hypothetical and have been extrapolated from actual state cancer registry data for a population of 3.5 to 4 million residents.

38 percent and 40 percent for 1998–1999 and 2000–2001, respectively. Although slightly higher, those rates were in line with the national trend. Consistent with the national trends, black and Hispanic males had higher rates than non-Hispanic white males. In some counties, those differences are quite large.

Gary had photocopies of a table and two charts published in the same issue of *Cancer Facts and Figures* that Archie had referred to earlier. The graphics tell an important story for the state because the state and national rates are so similar. "Here's what these data tell us," Gary said. "First, national results from the Behavioral Risk Factor Surveillance System (Table 2.3) clearly indicate that screening for colorectal cancer is low. Second, among those who have been screened and found to be positive, only 37% were found to have localized disease (Figure 2.1). Finally, we can see that survival rates are

TABLE 2.3 Colon and Rectum Screening, Adults 50 and Older, United States, 1999*

%	Recent Fecal Occult Blood Test[†]			% Recent Sigmoidoscopy/ Colonoscopy[‡]		
	Total %	Male %	Female %	Total %	Male %	Female %
Age						
50–59	15.6	13.4	17.6	26.2	28.8	23.8
60–69	23.3	21.4	24.8	37.2	41.9	33.4
70–79	26.0	25.1	26.6	40.9	45.7	37.5
80–84	24.0	22.8	24.7	39.1	47.8	34.5
85+	17.3	16.0	17.9	30.6	33.9	29.2
Race/Ethnicity						
White	21.2	19.4	22.7	33.9	37.3	31.1
Black	20.5	17.7	22.6	32.8	38.3	28.9
Asian/Pacific Islander	8.8	7.5	10.4	31.4	38.8	21.9
American Indian/ Alaska Native	17.6	13.6	21.2	34.0	31.7	36.3
Hispanic	11.7	10.9	12.3	29.5	31.4	27.9
Non-Hispanic	21.5	19.4	23.1	34.0	37.7	31.0

*Includes the 50 states and the District of Columbia.
[†]A fecal occult blood test within the last year.
[‡]A sigmoidoscopy or colonoscopy within the preceding five years.
Source: Behavioral Risk Factor Surveillance System CD-ROM 1999, National Center for Disease Prevention and Health Promotion, Centers for Disease Control and Prevention, 2000.

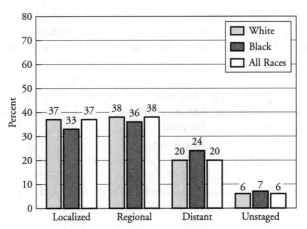

FIGURE 2.1   Percent Colorectal Cancer Cases Diagnosed
by Stage and Race, United States, 1992–1997
*Rates are based on the follow-up of patients through 1997.
Source: SEER Cancer Statistics Review, 1973–1998,
Surveillance, Epidemiology, and End Results Program, Division of
Cancer Control and Population Sciences, National Cancer
Institute, 2001.

substantially higher if the disease is detected when it is still localized (Figure 2.2). So, I think this gives us some pretty compelling evidence that there are some gaps that sound prevention programs can close."

Gary paused and started looking through his briefcase. "Here it is—a report from CDC I thought might be helpful. It presents data indicating that screening prevalence rates are especially low among people who are 50–64 years old, have low income, little or no health insurance, and limited education. Our state data say the same thing!"

The First Draft

Elaine Elkins turned in the last of the completed interviews one week later. The feedback confirmed what Archie had expected. The local health districts thought the breast and cervical cancer prevention effort had gone well and offered a good base to build on. The districts also wanted "flexibility." They didn't want to be limited to addressing a few "categorical" cancers to the exclusion of others. Respondents pointed out that things changed quickly, and they needed support to anticipate and address those changes as they arose. For example, in one district, dentists had been quite vocal about the use of smokeless tobacco. Results from the 2001 Youth Risk Behavior Survey

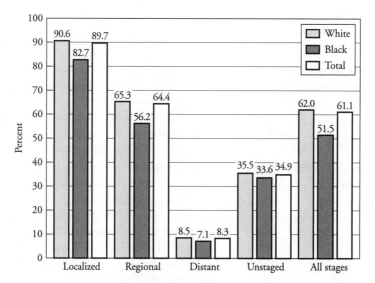

**FIGURE 2.2   Five-Year Survival Rates by Stage at Diagnosis
and Race, 1992–1997**

Rates are based on the population-based registries in Connecticut, New Mexico,
Iowa, Hawaii, Atlanta, Detroit Seattle–Puget Sound, and San Francisco–
Oakland. Rates are based on follow-up of patients through 1997.
Source: SEER Cancer Statistics Review, 1973–1998, Surveillance, Epidemiology,
and End Results Program, Division of Cancer Control and Population Sciences,
National Cancer Institute, 2001.

(YRBS) carried out in the county high schools indicated that 22 percent of
boys in grades 9–12 reported using chewing tobacco or snuff on one or more
occasions in the past 30 days, more than double the state rate.

In summary, the results of the telephone surveys with the local health
officers would give the proposal a "local voice," reinforcing the need to move
in a more comprehensive direction and to build on their prior accomplishments. Based on the assessment of state and national data that Gary Lee provided and on the results of the interviews, Archie crafted an interpretation of
"a comprehensive approach to prevention." Table 2.4 shows the characteristics of his comprehensive approach, with examples.

A short time after Archie had come to his insight about what a *comprehensive* approach might mean, Gary e-mailed him an attachment containing
information he had picked up during his trip to Atlanta. CDC was apparently moving fast toward the development of a grant program to states supporting what it was calling a comprehensive approach to cancer control. Gary
included a diagram of the framework used by CDC (Figure 2.3).

TABLE 2.4 Characteristics and Examples of a "Comprehensive" Approach

Characteristic	Example
Goes beyond addressing one health problem at a time	Seven health districts in the state document the need to address at least three different cancer prevention and control strategies. Each will be eligible for support because resources are not restricted to a categorical cancer problem.
Takes action after assessing connections among health problems as well as among their respective risk factors	Many cancers are linked through just a few risk factors. Furthermore, those risk factors are themselves closely connected, as with nutrition and physical activity or alcohol and sexual activity. Districts can combine resources from separate disease funds to mount more effective efforts that address clusters of related risks.
Is flexible enough to match the unique conditions of each community	Different districts face different challenges in assuring the *local conditions* for effective cancer prevention. For example, obstacles to physical activity are different for people in sprawling suburbs versus those in migrant worker camps. Even as communities focus on the same risk factors, each will have the latitude to decide for itself how to use local assets and strengths in directing local forces of change.
Complements categorical programs	The heaviest burden of cancer, by far, is borne by just a few subgroups in each district: ethnic minorities, people with low income, and people exposed to workplace or environmental hazards. Beyond cancer, those same people have the highest rates of other health problems along with the worst housing, education, and economic opportunities. Investments that improve the basic living conditions in communities will reinforce not only cancer prevention, but also health and human development across the board.

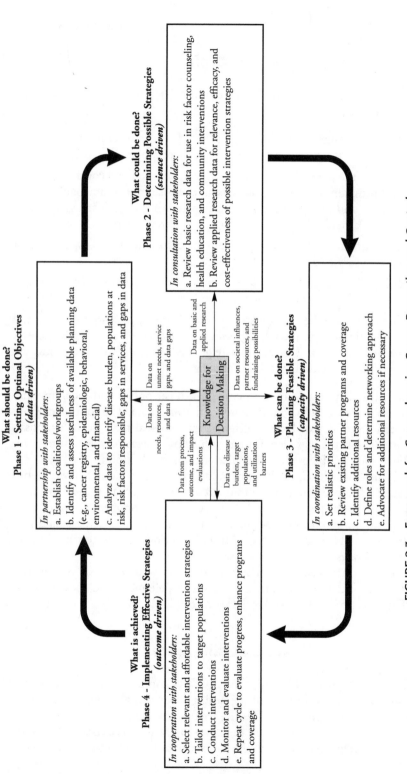

FIGURE 2.3   Framework for Comprehensive Cancer Prevention and Control

Source: Abed J, Reilley B, Odell Butler M, Kean T, Wong F, Hohman K. Developing a framework for comprehensive cancer prevention and control in the United States: an initiative of the Centers for Disease Control and Prevention. *Journal of Public Health Management and Practice.* 2000;6(2):70.

The Draft

Archie's draft proposal was well crafted and brief (15 pages), and its salient features stood out:

- It was built upon the achievements and the infrastructure that had been created by the good work of existing cancer programs.
- It made the point that effective cancer prevention and control planning and programming should address all of those cancers amenable to prevention and early detection, yet recognized the unique challenges found among different population groups in different parts of the state.
- It documented the need to address the disparities that exist because of gaps in service delivery and coverage.
- It highlighted the importance of involving a wide variety of stakeholders, especially at the local level.
- It emphasized the need to strengthen the state's capacity to review and use epidemiological data, including data collected by the state central cancer registry and survey data (e.g., BRFSS and YBRS) to jointly set priorities for action and monitor progress.

Archie had taken great care to document critical points and recommendations with evidence from county, state, or national data. The comments from the telephone survey of local health districts put real faces in the proposal.

Archie left the completed draft with Judith's secretary, Jean Turner, on the 28th, two days before his scheduled meeting with Judith.

As she read the draft, Judith couldn't hide her pleasure. It was better than she had hoped for, and she told Archie precisely that at their meeting. They discussed the paper and Judith made several recommendations, mostly about positioning of certain issues. The two decided that Archie would present his proposal as a report at a special staff meeting that Judith would call in the next few days.

At the staff meeting, Archie's report was well received. Afterwards, Judith assembled a team to cost out the various elements and craft the budget. The final proposal got to Dr. Jackson's office on time.

Four Months Later

Just as Dr. Westphal had hoped, the HPCDP's comprehensive cancer initiative emerged as a top priority for the health department in its budget recommendations to the governor. The hard work of Archie Graham and other HPCDP staffers had paid off, but there was little time to celebrate. When the governor's budget bill reached the appropriations committee, the health department's proposed new initiatives became an important issue. The committee wanted further explanation of the projects and called for testimony from the health department director, Dr. Joseph Jackson.

At 8 a.m. on the morning Dr. Jackson was scheduled to testify, his wife called the health department to tell his staff that he had been stricken with the flu and would not be able to meet with the appropriations committee as planned. Dr. Jackson asked that Dr. Westphal serve in his capacity before the committee. At 8:15, Judith was informed that she was to fill in for Dr. Jackson at the 10:30 meeting at the capitol. She immediately contacted Archie Graham and explained that she wanted him to accompany her to the meeting for backup in the event that the committee asked questions requiring interpretation of the data upon which the initiative was based.

Following Judith's testimony, the committee chair, Representative Leo Mazzone, a long-time advocate of public programs for the economically disadvantaged, questioned the importance of the new initiative.

"Dr. Westphal, thank you for taking time out of your busy day to testify before this committee," he began. "It is clear that your people have put a good deal of time and effort into this proposal."

Representative Mazzone removed his glasses and rubbed his eyes before continuing. "As much as I support the philosophy of prevention, I have a hard time seeing this program as a state priority when we are faced with other pressing issues like the crisis in our emergency rooms—right here in this city they are overcrowded, underfunded, and so full they routinely turn ambulances away. The media are full of stories about it. Shouldn't this be a priority?"

Archie squirmed in his chair and thought to himself, "Here we go again, treatment versus prevention."

Judith's response was measured and respectful. "Representative Mazzone, my brother is an emergency room physician and I can confirm that overcrowding is a growing problem. Too often, those without access to regular care turn to emergency rooms for routine health care needs and that care is expensive. As we pointed out in the proposal, our comprehensive cancer program will provide screening and preventive services for all residents statewide, with special emphasis on those with low incomes and those who are uninsured. A statewide comprehensive program of prevention will contribute to reducing the burden on emergency rooms."

Representative Mazzone nodded and asked whether the committee members had any further questions for Dr. Westphal before she was dismissed. Vard Maxwell, the most senior member of the committee, gestured to the chairman and leaned forward in his seat. He cleared his throat and sipped from a cup of water. "Mr. Chairman, this is not so much a question for Dr. Westphal as it is a comment to my colleagues on this committee," he said. "As most of you know, my wife, Nita, is a survivor of breast cancer. She's 65 years old and has lived five happy and productive years since her diagnosis and surgery. I hope and expect she's going to be around for many more, too."

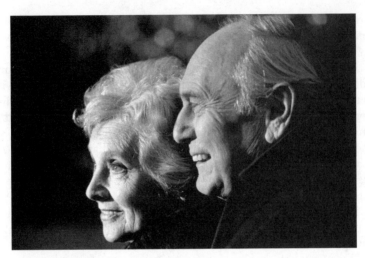

Vard and Nita Maxwell

He continued, "But I'm smart enough to realize that Nita's here today because she's got private insurance and a wonderful physician, and she had regular mammograms. Her cancer was detected early, when it could still be treated effectively. Not all women have that benefit. Nor do men. But they ought to. The high rates of colorectal cancer, especially among black and Hispanic males, we heard about today are embarrassing." He eased back in his chair. "I think this is precisely the kind of program we should support."

Judith smiled kindly at Representative Maxwell. Archie looked down at his notepad. The committee remained silent until the chairman spoke. "Thank you for coming today, Dr. Westphal, Mr. Graham," he said. "We appreciate your time."

Case Analysis

Judith and Archie were fortunate that Vard Maxwell added such a compelling personal note to their presentation. However, the success of their presentation can be attributed to more than luck. Judith's sound management skills set the stage with the right questions. She anticipated the upcoming task and gave her staff enough lead time to do a thorough job. She also delegated tasks, with appropriate guidance, to Archie. Archie, in turn, sought input from several sources to build a solid case. He applied his own technical skills to translate the resulting data into a coherent proposal.

In this section, we provide some additional information and examples of how to obtain and use data—the two tasks that Judith and Archie performed so well and that lie at the heart of effective public health practice.

TYPES AND SOURCES OF PUBLIC HEALTH DATA

The first step in identifying sources of information is to find out what is readily available within your organization. This may seem like an obvious suggestion, but in many large agencies (and some smaller ones, too), a wide variety of useful information sits in computers or on shelves, unbeknownst to those who might find it helpful. Annual reports, legislative testimony, and other policy documents often provide compilations of relevant data.

Helpful Resources and Models

Since the late 1980s, CDC has developed, in close coordination with the National Association of County and City Health Officials (NACCHO), a series of protocols designed to enhance the development of community health improvement programs. While reading about them may trigger visions of alphabet soup, practitioners who apply their principles and methods will find them most helpful. Among the most notable early iterations were the Planned Approach to Community Health (PATCH) and the Assessment Protocol for Excellence in Public Health (APEX/PH). The most recent and advanced version, Mobilizing for Action through Planning and Partnerships (MAPP), is a communitywide strategic planning tool for improving community health.[7] Facilitated by public health leadership, this tool helps communities prioritize public health issues and identify resources for addressing them.

Consistent with the approach employed by PATCH and APEX/PH, community ownership is the fundamental component of MAPP. Because the community's strengths, needs, and desires drive the process, MAPP provides a framework for creating a community-driven initiative. Archie's commitment to eliciting input from the local health districts community was a manifestation of his understanding that participation leads to collective thinking and ultimately results in programs that are effective and accountable.

Community participation is essential for another reason. Health departments cannot act alone; it takes a wide range of organizations and individuals to contribute to the public's health. Public, private, and voluntary organizations bring community members together, and even informal associations have a major role to play in public health improvement. The MAPP process brings these diverse interests together to collaboratively determine the most effective way to conduct public health activities. This important concept is reiterated in Chapter 5 in the description and discussion of the theory of social capital.

To initiate the MAPP process, lead organizations in the community begin by organizing themselves and preparing to implement MAPP. Communitywide strategic planning requires a high level of commitment from partners, stakeholders, and the community residents who are recruited to participate.

The MAPP protocol guides users through four levels of assessments:

- The ***Community Themes and Strength Assessment*** provides a deep understanding of the issues residents feel are important by answering the questions *"What is important to our community?" "How is quality of life perceived in our community?"* and *"What assets do we have that can be used to improve community health?"*

- The ***Local Public Health System Assessment (LPHSA)*** is a comprehensive assessment of all of the organizations and entities that contribute to the public's health. The LPHSA answers the questions *"What are the activities, competencies, and capacities of our local public health system?"* and *"How are the essential services being provided to our community?"*

- The ***Community Health Status Assessment (CHSA)*** identifies high-priority issues related to community health and quality of life. Questions answered during the phase include *"How healthy are our residents?"* and *"What does the health status of our community look like?"*

  Data indicators that can provide answers to those questions include:

  1. Demographic characteristics
  2. Socioeconomic characteristics
  3. Health resource availability
  4. Quality of life
  5. Behavioral risk factors
  6. Environmental indicators
  7. Social and mental health
  8. Maternal and child health
  9. Death, illness, and injury
  10. Infectious disease
  11. Sentinel events

- The ***Forces of Change Assessment*** identifies forces such as legislation, technology, and other issues that affect the context in which the community and its public health system operate. It answers the questions *"What is occurring or might occur that affects the health of our community or the local public health system?"* and *"What specific threats or opportunities are generated by these occurrences?"*

With good baseline data in hand, the MAPP process guides you through a series of six steps.

Step 1: Prepare for the Community

A subcommittee should be designated to oversee the process. Members should include individuals who can assist with access to data as well as data collection, analysis, and interpretation. Community representatives also provide an important perspective. Once the subcommittee is assembled, members should review the CHSA steps and identify the skills and resources needed to conduct the activities.

Step 2: Collect Data for the Core Indicators

During this step, data related to the MAPP "core indicators" should be collected, including trend and comparison data. Trend data will help to identify changes in data over time, while comparison data will measure a community's health status against that of other jurisdictions. Data collection may require considerable time and effort, so it is important to begin this activity early in the MAPP process.

Step 3: Identify Locally Appropriate Indicators and Collect Data

The selection of locally appropriate indicators helps the MAPP Committee better describe the community's health status and quality of life in terms that are of particular interest to the community. Additional indicators might be selected that relate to community interest in a specific topic, demographics in the area (e.g., an aging population), or information found in the core indicators (e.g., the need to look more closely at cancer rates). To keep data collection efforts reasonable in terms of time and resources, select indicators of high priority and relevance only.

Step 4: Organize and Analyze Data, Compile the Findings, and Disseminate the Information

Individuals with statistical expertise should analyze data. Disparities among age, gender, racial, and other population subgroups are especially important. Once the data are analyzed, a compilation of the findings or a "community health profile" should be developed. The community health profile should include visual aids, such as charts and graphs, that display the data in an understandable and meaningful way. The community health profile should be disseminated and shared with the community.

Step 5: Establish a System to Monitor Indicators over Time

During this step, the committee establishes a system for monitoring selected indicators. This effort helps to ensure that continuous health status monitoring occurs and establishes baseline data upon which future trends can be identified. This system will also be instrumental in evaluating the success of MAPP activities.

Step 6: Identify Challenges and Opportunities Related to Health Status

The assessment process should result in a list of challenges and opportunities related to the community's health status. Data findings should be reviewed to identify challenges, such as major health problems or high-risk behaviors, and opportunities, such as improving health trends. Ideally, the final list will include 10–15 community health status issues that will be more closely examined in the strategic issues identification phase of MAPP.

Finding Data

Mortality data are generally tracked by vital statistics departments, which also record births, marriages, and divorces. In some states, vital statistics departments are part of the health department. All 50 states collect mortality data in a standardized format, and some capture additional information (such as smoking status). Each state's information is reported to CDC's National Center for Health Statistics (NCHS), which compiles a national data set. (Access to national mortality data sets is discussed later.)

Mortality data sets include demographic information on the deceased, plus where he or she lived and died, whether the death occurred in a hospital or institution, and what caused his or her death. The cause of death is translated into a medical code described in the *Manual of the International Statistical Classification of Diseases, Injuries, and Causes of Death,* ninth revision (the ICD-9 code). The tenth revision, ICD-10, is expected to be available by the end of 2003.

Hospital discharge data are available in most states and can be a useful tool for determining public health problems as well as treatment patterns, access to care, and costs associated with various diseases or procedures. Data sets typically include age, race, sex, area of residence, year of discharge, length of hospital stay, and diagnoses.

Hospital discharge data are not always found in vital statistics departments; they may be under the purview of insurance departments or governor's-level commissions. The extent to which these data are made available to public health practitioners varies widely, and restrictions are common to protect individuals' privacy. Even when hospital discharge data are available, they may not cover all hospitals in a given area. Practitioners will find state epidemiologists a great resource for accessing and interpreting these data for program planning.

Behavioral risk factors offer important insights into the lifestyle choices that are such stubborn contributors to poor health outcomes. They are tracked through a monthly CDC telephone survey of adults, called the *Behavioral Risk Factors Surveillance System (BRFSS)*. BRFSS is now in place in every state. Over an 8- to 14-day period, telephone survey staff in each state conduct between 100 and 300 interviews. A set of core questions has been used consistently since the survey was introduced in 1981. These questions cover physical activity, blood pressure, diet, body weight, smoking, alcohol consumption, and use of preventive services. The CDC also develops modules on specific topics (such as breast and cervical cancer screening or smoke detector use) that states may opt to include. States have the option of adding state-specific questions of particular interest to them. Since 1993, the surveys have retained the core questions and rotated additional questions every year.

Traditionally, the BRFSS yields state-level data. Therefore, those data can serve only as an imprecise estimate of what is occurring in a given locality. However, in several states, concerted efforts are being made to oversample certain areas so as to provide valid and reliable local-level estimates. Over time, more states have moved in that direction.

CDC, working through state health and education agencies, also supports two school-based surveillance systems. The *Youth Risk Behavior Surveillance System (YRBSS)* provides similar information for a wide range of health indicators relevant to high-school-age youth. The *Youth Tobacco Survey (YTS)* provides state-based data on students' knowledge, attitudes, and behaviors related to tobacco use. It also assesses cessation behavior, media awareness, and exposure to environmental tobacco smoke.

By definition, **national data** comprise information gathered from national surveys or from compilations of data submitted by states and localities. For example, state and local health departments in your area may already participate in data collection geared toward national indicators such as *Healthy People 2010: National Health Promotion and Disease Prevention Objectives.*[8] For local practitioners, national data are most often used to illustrate national trends or as a point of reference against which one can compare the local situation. Recall that Gary Lee drew Archie Graham's attention to the importance of comparing county and state cancer data to national trends.

National indicators can also help you frame the unit of measurement for a particular health problem. For example, if you were interested in improving nutrition among a particular population, which indicators would tell you that you were making progress? According to *Healthy People 2010,* you would want to track dietary fat intake, calcium intake, breast-feeding, nutrition labeling, the availability of reduced-fat processed foods, and nutrition assessments and referrals by clinicians, among many other indicators. You might also come up with other indicators relevant to your community or program. In any case, these indicators can be a good starting point—especially for a disease or risk factor that is new to you.

CDC collects, maintains, and disseminates vast amounts of health-related data. Indeed, coordinating the nation's surveillance system is one of the agency's most important and long-standing contributions to public health. Furthermore, modifications and updates to these systems, as well as innovations, occur regularly.

The National Center for Health Statistics (NCHS) is part of CDC. Its mission is to support state and local health departments as they try to increase their capacity to analyze and use data for public health policy development and program management, particularly as related to health promotion. NCHS emphasizes the importance of establishing a sustainable statistical capacity in all states and provides technical assistance to state and local health agencies in support of that goal.

Fortunately, technological advances have made products from CDC and NCHS readily accessible to anyone with a computer and a modem. For rapid access to national health statistics, we would encourage health promotion practitioners to periodically search the NCHS and CDC Web sites and the links to the sites of their collaborating domestic and international partners.[9]

Clearly, public health has moved far beyond its former confines of communicable disease control. The attention now paid to lifestyle and behaviors as risk factors for a wide variety of diseases and conditions is just one example of its expansion. Indeed, public health's dual focus on individual and community health brings an even wider scope of problems into view, many of which do not fall within the traditional confines of public health. For example, in most communities, violence and motor vehicle injuries are heavy contributors to morbidity and mortality. Understanding their toll on communities and designing interventions to reduce that toll requires interaction with numerous other agencies—law enforcement, criminal justice, education, and traffic safety, among others. These agencies offer combinations of national, state, and local data sets that are comparable to those for health indicators discussed earlier. For example, the National Highway Traffic Safety Administration maintains the Fatal Accident Reporting System (FARS), which is based on state and local data reported from police investigations of automobile crash sites. The National Institute of Justice maintains a drugs and crime data center that provides statistics and publications.

There has been no more dramatic example of the need for interorganizational collaboration than the drive to establish the local capacity for bioterrorism preparedness and response. Such action requires the close collaboration of virtually every sector of society: law, safety, health, education, travel, communications, fire transportation, and so on. In planning such a complex activity, each of the collaborating partners will have to bring its respective databases and insights to the table and be prepared to share them in a way that is understandable to all.

People: Experience, Perception, and Wisdom

Understandably, research reports and journal articles, grounded in credible science, serve as primary sources of knowledge and insight for health promotion practitioners. Nevertheless, philosopher Ken Wilber[10] confirms what common sense tells us—there are different ways of knowing and different interpretations of "reality." Participatory research in public health has taught us that an epidemiologist, an anthropologist, a health educator, and a layperson are likely to view a given problem through different lenses. More importantly, each is quite likely to detect a glimpse of reality that the others may miss.

That said, the wisdom that comes from experience can add rich contributions and insight to the quantitative evidence one gathers to plan or justify health promotion actions. Recall Judith Westphal's directions, Gary Lee's insights on data, the input from local health district directors—all of this "wisdom and insight" helped point Archie Graham in the right direction and undoubtedly had a direct impact on the quality of his proposal.

Seek out the wisdom of others; take advantage of what they have experienced. How often have we read through articles or reports about an effective intervention program, only to discover that the description of the methods used is cursory at best? Most journals want authors to emphasize their data-based findings—they are less interested in detailed accounts of what actually took place. Take the time to try to contact the author by e-mail or phone. If authors don't have enough time to talk to you, they will tell you so, and you will be no worse off. However, if you give them the courtesy of some preparation and thinking ahead of time, chances are they'll help you or provide you with the contact information of someone who can.

A Cautionary Note

Within reason, using a variety of sources and portrayals of information will help you develop a richer, more nuanced description of any given problem. Data on public health problems reflect the complexity and interrelated nature of the problems themselves. We rarely see a clean, unbroken line between cause and effect, nor do we have the luxury of consulting a recent survey that polled the exact population we're interested in about the exact behavior we want to modify. Instead, we typically find ourselves trying to disentangle a knot of behaviors, socioeconomic conditions, susceptibility to disease, and sheer chance. Some data may contradict each other, or fall short in terms of comprehensiveness, or seem out of date—among many other drawbacks.

These data problems don't necessarily have to be solved, but they do have to be acknowledged in your assumptions and in your portrayals and uses of data. For example, we don't know the true homeless population in the community because, among other census problems, estimates cannot capture the number of people who are doubled up in friends' and relatives' apartments because they cannot afford their own. When we explain why we have designed a health care program for the homeless based on larger estimates of need than the documented homeless population, this is one of the reasons. As you inform yourself about the health problem you are trying to address, keep track of gaps in your data and note how they affect your intervention and its evaluation.

USING LOCAL DATA TO STIMULATE LOCAL ACTION

Globally we have observed a steady increase in the number of communities that have formed alliances or partnerships for the purpose of health promotion. This collaborative movement has certainly been influenced by a wide range of initiatives sharing a common goal. MAPP, referenced earlier in this chapter, is one recent example. Others include the Planned Approach to Community Health (PATCH), Healthy Cities, Sustainable Communities and the Center for Civic Partnerships, Healthy Communities, and an initiative called *Turning Point*. Actually, the full title of the latter effort is *Turning Point: Collaborating for a New Century in Public Health*. It is sponsored by the Robert Wood Johnson Foundation and W. K. Kellogg Foundation and is directed by the School of Public Health, University of Washington, in collaboration with the National Association of County and City Health Officials (NACCHO). As of January 2003, *Turning Point* had established 21 state-level partnerships and 41 partnerships in communities and tribal jurisdictions across those states.

We highlight *Turning Point* here because its mission and purpose capture the principles and values shared by many of the other initiatives that make up the community collaborative movement to promote health. Paraphrased, its mission statement is as follows:

> To transform and strengthen the current public health system so that states, communities, and their public health agencies may respond to the challenge to protect and improve the public's health in the 21st century . . . this mission is achieved by the creation of a safe learning environment where **local communities, state agencies, and their partners can work collaboratively to analyze and address significant challenges** pertaining to public health system improvements . . . the challenges include, but are not limited to, **workforce development and deployment**; establishing and sustaining community linkages; **eliminating health disparities**; assuring access to quality care; and **increasing public awareness of and participation** in public health activity.

The boldfaced phrases highlight some of the common values shared by community collaborative initiatives: (1) state and local partners working collaboratively to analyze and address challenges, (2) envisioning "health" in a broad sense so that issues such as employment and health disparities constitute legitimate points of intervention, and (3) engaging the public and enhancing their awareness. The logic is straightforward and goes something like this: Health improvement requires complex changes; complex changes are more likely to be supported by citizens who are informed about and embrace the need for those changes.

Local Use of Data

A clear manifestation of this logic can be seen in the following examples of how local data on different indicators are being creatively translated to heighten public concern for, and interest in, a community's health improvement.

The 1995 North Carolina Report Card for the state's Child Health Day (Figure 2.4) was prepared by the North Carolina Institute of Medicine in collaboration with the Division of Maternal and Child Health within the Department of Environment, Health, and Natural Resources; the North Carolina Pediatric Society; and the state's Area Health Education Centers. The report card's authors selected health indicators in 19 categories deemed relevant to the health of children and adolescents, ranging from child abuse and maltreatment to teen pregnancies, injuries, and immunization rates. For each indicator, the report card shows where North Carolina stood in 1993 or 1994 (the most recent years for which data were available) and how these levels compared to state and/or national goals for 2000. Grades were assigned for each indicator, depending on the size of the gap between current indicators and the 2000 goals. The overall message from these comparisons is prominently displayed on the front cover of the report card: "C-minus—We can do better!"

The Community Benchmarking Collaborative is a joint project of the Berkeley–Charleston–Dorchester Council of Governments, the Chamber of Commerce, and several other philanthropic organizations serving coastal South Carolina. This regional collaborative effort developed a document called *Measuring for Success 2000.* It was intended to serve as a visible and reliable source of information about the quality of life in the Berkeley–Charleston–Dorchester counties in South Carolina. Patterned after similar studies conducted throughout the country, the project's purpose is to measure the Tri-County region's progress in advancing the quality of life.

Each year, the Benchmarking Collaborative partners collect, analyze, and monitor data about major areas of the region and report their results. Their goal is to use selected indicators to heighten public knowledge about the region's quality of life in the hope that greater awareness will stimulate action to address the challenges and opportunities emerging in their region. The group's commitment is to produce the report every year through 2010.

In *Measuring for Success 2001,* the collaborative chose to address 11 topic areas: the region's population, measures of poverty, jobs and wages, the housing market, a healthy start, preparing for our future, natural environment, transportation systems, a safe place, race relations, and public mood. Note that only two categories (a healthy start and a safe place) constitute what might be referred to as traditional health indicators. More and

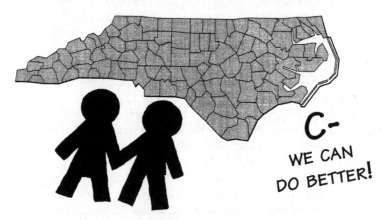

1995
North Carolina
<u>Report Card</u>

CHILD HEALTH DAY

C-
WE CAN
DO BETTER!

OCTOBER 2nd

NORTH CAROLINA INSTITUTE OF MEDICINE

Citizens dedicated to improving the health of North Carolinians

DEHNR
NC Division of Maternal & Child Health,
Department of Environment, Health
and Natural Resources

NORTH CAROLINA
PEDIATRIC SOCIETY

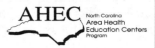
AHEC
North Carolina
Area Health
Education Centers
Program

In collaboration with The American Health Foundation, New York, NY

FIGURE 2.4   North Carolina Child Health Report Card

(figure continues through page 46)

HEALTH INDICATOR:	Year	NC Data	Target for Year 2000[16,17]	Grade
Immunization Rates				
% of children under 2 years with basic series completed[6]	1991	64.9	NC Goal: 90.0	B-
% of children with basic series completed at school entry[6]	1994	98	NC Goal: 98.0	A
Vaccine-Preventable Diseases (# cases ages 0-19)[7]				
Measles	1994	3	US Goal: 0	A-
Mumps	1994	73	US Goal: 0	C
Rubella	1994	0	US Goal: 0	A
Diphtheria	1994	0	US Goal: 0	A
Pertussis	1994	140	US Goal: 1,000 cases	C
Tetanus	1994	0	US Goal: 0	A
Polio	1994	0	US Goal: 0	A
Hepatitis B, # of cases per 100,000 population	1994	4.1	US Goal: 9.4	A
Hemophilus influenza, Type B	1994	32		B
Dental Disease				
Sealants: % of children with one or more sealants, 5th and 6th graders[8]	1994	23	NC Goal: 50; US Goal: 50	C-
% of children on fluoridated water systems[8]	1994	78		C+
Environmental Health				
% of preschool children screened for lead levels[9]	1994	15	NC Goal: 40.0	D
% of screened children with elevated blood lead ($\geq15\mu g/dl$), ages 6 months to 6 years[9]	10/92-9/94	2.5	US Goal: 2.0	C
Head Start				
% of eligible 3 and 4 year olds enrolled[10]	1994-95	31.9		C

HEALTH INDICATOR:	Year	NC Data	Target for Year 2000[16,17]	Grade
Alcohol, Tobacco and Substance Abuse				
Cigarette Smoking				
% daily smokers, grades 11-12[1]	1993	21.0	NC Goal: 9.0	D
Smokeless Tobacco Use				
% using in past 30 days, grades 11-12[1]	1993	11.7	NC Goal: 4.0	D
Marijuana Use				
% using in past 30 days, grades 11-12[1]	1993	15.0	NC Goal: 8.0	D
Alcohol				
% of students grades 11-12 who drank beer in past 30 days[1]	1993	44.0	NC Goal: 17.0	D
Cocaine				
% of students who said they used in past month[2]	1993	2.0		D
Asthma				
# of hospital discharges per 10,000 population, ages 0-14[3]	1992	24.5	US Goal: less than 30 per 10,000	A
Child Abuse and Maltreatment				
Number of cases[4]	1994	18,397	NC Goal: 22,274	B-
Child Sexual Abuse				
Number of cases[1]	1993	1,447	NC Goal: 1,365	B-
Communicable Diseases				
# of syphilis, gonorrhea, chlamydia cases, ages 15-24[1]	1993	28,407	NC Goal: 23,968	B-
# of reported cases of children, ages 0-9, with AIDS[5]	1993	7		C

FIGURE 2.4 *continued*

HEALTH INDICATOR:	Year	NC Data	Target for Year 2000[16,17]	Grade
Infant Mortality[11]				
Total # deaths/1,000 live births	1994	10.0	NC Goal: 7.4; US Goal: 7.0	C
Non-white	1994	15.6	NC Goal: 8.7 US Goal for African Americans: 11.0	D
% Low Birth Weight (5.5 lbs. or less)[11]				
Total	1994	8.7	NC Goal: 7.0; US Goal: 5.0	B
Non-White	1994	13.1	NC Goal: 10.4 US Goal for African Americans: 9.0	C
Teen Pregnancies (ages 15-17/1,000 girls in age group)[1]				
Total	1993	62.4	NC Goal: 63.0 US Goal: 50	A -
Non-White	1993	110.7	NC Goal: 86.7	B -
Prenatal Care (% of mothers aged 10-19 having LATE or NO PRENATAL CARE)[12]				
Total	1988-92	44.5		C
White	1988-92	37.1		C
Minorities	1988-92	52.3		D+
% of Live Births with NO PRENATAL CARE, Mothers' Ages 10-17[13]				
Total	1992	29		C
White	1992	1.9		C
Non-White	1992	37		C

HEALTH INDICATOR:	Year	NC Data	Target for Year 2000[16,17]	Grade
Injuries				
Unintentional				
Motor vehicle death rate, ages 15-24[1]	1991-93	33.6	NC Goal: 29.6	C
# of drowning deaths, ages 0-19[14]	1993	56		C
Fires/Burns, # of deaths, ages 0-19[14]	1993	20		C
Poisoning, # of deaths, ages 0-19[14]	1993	4		C
Intentional (# of deaths)				
Suicide, ages 0-19[14]	1993	61		C -
Homicide, ages 0-19[14]	1993	135		C -
Firearms, ages 0-19[14]	1993	161		C -
Early intervention to reduce effects of developmental delay, emotional disturbance, and/or chronic illness[15]	1994	6,104	NC Goal: 8,000	B
Nutrition[1]				
% Overweight:				
Low income children ages 0-4	1992	7.1	NC Goal: 5.0	C
Low income children ages 5-11	1992	17.1	NC Goal: 10.0	D
Persons 12-19	1992	40	NC Goal: 15.0; US Goal: 15.0	D
Physical Fitness[2]				
% of all high school students with physical education classes during an average school week	1993	47		C

FIGURE 2.4 *continued*

more people are coming to the realization that social, economic, and cultural determinants are key factors in determining quality of life and health in their community. Figures 2.5 and 2.6 show responses to selected questions from the survey about race relations in the Tri-County region. Data like these make

In the past year, have you or anyone in you household experienced discrimination?

(If yes), as I read from the following list, please tell me what the discrimination was based on:

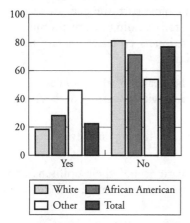

	White	African American	Other	Total
Age	17.4	0	0	9.4
Disability or handicap	4.3	3.8	0	3.5
Gender	19.6	0	15.4	12.9
Other	8.7	15.4	7.7	10.6
Race	37.1	76.9	76.9	56.5
Religion	2.2	0	0	1.2
Sexual orientation	8.7	3.8	0	5.9

FIGURE 2.5   Findings Related to "Experiencing" Discrimination, 2000
Source: Measuring for Success 2001: A Study of the Issues That Will Shape Our Region.
Charleston, SC: Community Benchmarking Collaborative, Charleston Metro Chamber of
Commerce; 2001:22.

Do you think racial discrimination is a problem in the Tri-County area?

(If yes), is racial discrimination greatest in the area of:

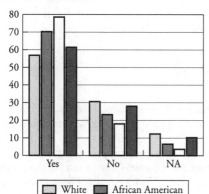

	White	African American	Other	Total
Education	20.3	19.4	10.0	19.1
Employment	28.4	40.3	55.0	33.9
Housing	18.9	12.9	10.0	16.5
Politics	17.6	17.7	5.0	16.5
Other	14.9	9.7	20.0	13.9

FIGURE 2.6   Findings Related to Discrimination as a "Problem," 2000
Source: Measuring for Success 2001: A Study of the Issues That Will Shape Our Region.
Charleston, SC: Community Benchmarking Collaborative, Charleston Metro Chamber of
Commerce; 2001:22–23.

it difficult for planners to ignore the important role that social factors (in this case, discrimination) play in influencing the quality of life of a community.

SUMMARY

In this chapter, we have pointed out that health-related data constitute a critical source of knowledge for planners. For the most part, the data are readily available and accessible to those responsible for planning health promotion programs. Effective health promotion practitioners typically operate using three assumptions about such health-related data:

1. In the absence of relevant data about the health of the population we serve, we cannot set priorities, plan programs with precision, or determine how or whether those programs work.

2. We must know what questions to ask before, during, and even after the data-collection process.

3. People are an essential source of information, and their opinions and views should be actively sought out, respected, and integrated into the decision-making process.

We have used numerous examples of data in this chapter to familiarize readers with the vast body of health information sources that are available and accessible in the field. In so doing, we recognize that some may interpret this to be akin to data collection "overkill." Our position is simply this: Responsible planners need to be aware of where the data sources are and know how to inquire about the relevance of those data to their various health promotion tasks. Somewhere between the extremes of operating on intuition and no information on the one hand, and the paralysis that results from having mounds of data on the other, lies the prudent middle ground.

ENDNOTES

1. While our description follows the general process used by states in the United States, many of the same principles hold for provinces, states, and territories in other nations.
2. In the United States, state health agencies apply and compete for grants or cooperative agreements from the Centers for Disease Control and Prevention (CDC) or other U.S. Public Health Service (PHS) agencies. These grants are almost always tied to specific categories of health problems or issues such as cardiovascular disease, diabetes, injury prevention, obesity, HIV infection prevention, or asthma prevention and control.
3. There are 42 counties in the state that are divided into contiguous clusters, which in turn form 12 health districts.
4. Cancer Facts and Figures 2002. Atlanta: American Cancer Society; 2002:1.

5. McGinnis JM, Foege WH. Actual Causes of Death in the United States. *JAMA.* 1993;270(18):2207–2212.

6. Terms referencing ethnicity continue to be a source of considerable discussion and debate. In this case story, we have chosen to use the term "black" rather than "African American" because the data do not enable us to make the distinction between people of black color who may not be of African descent.

7. For more information about MAPP, contact the National Association of County and City Health Officials, 1100 17th Street, NW, Second Floor, Washington, DC 20036, phone: (202) 783-5550, e-mail: mapp@naccho.org.

8. U.S. Department of Health and Human Services. *Healthy People 2010: Objectives for the Nation.* Washington, DC: U.S. Government Printing Office; 2001.

9. The CDC Web site is http://www.cdc.gov; the direct Web site for NCHS is http://www.cdc.gov/nchs.

10. Wilber K. *Marriage of Sense and Soul: Integrating Science and Religion.* New York: Random House; 1998.

CHAPTER 3

Promoting Participation for Health

Case Story
THE COURT OF PUBLIC OPINION

It was nearly 6:30 p.m. and almost everyone had gone home an hour before. Ray Wycoff sat quietly at his desk, mindlessly elaborating on a series of circles he had sketched on the back of an envelope. It had been a long and frustrating day in what seemed to be a year's worth of long and frustrating days. The knock at the door startled him.

"Yes?"

The door opened slowly, leaving an opening large enough to frame the smiling face of Adam Solomon. "Planning to sleep over?"

Ray smiled. "What are you doing here?" In addition to being a neighbor and good friend, Adam Solomon was the managing editor for Hillsdale's daily paper, the *Sentinel-Dispatch,* and his office was located a block and a half from the Hillsdale Health Department.

"Hey, I'm a taxpayer and this is public property, isn't it?" Adam laughed. "I saw the light on in your office, and I need a ride home—the garage didn't have the parts in stock to fix my car so they had to keep it overnight."

Ray had always marveled at Adam, who at 34 was probably one of the youngest managing editors in the country. Although his work inevitably put him at the hub of political controversy, he was always on an even keel; his trademark was his irresistible sense of humor. Ray gestured toward the door as he got up. "Your taxi is waiting, sir!"

During the ride home, Ray was quiet and self-absorbed. "You look a little down," Adam observed. "What's up? Or down, as the case may be?"

Ray thought for a moment and then said, "Bottom line: I have come to the realization that I'm having a heck of a hard time doing the job I was hired to do and want to do!"

"You can't be serious!" Adam said, studying the expression on his friend's face. Then he added, "You are serious. What's going on?"

Ray didn't answer. He just pursed his lips and slowly shook his head from side to side. Adam knew that Ray's wife, Jeanne, had taken their two children to her mother's home in upstate New York. As Ray turned into

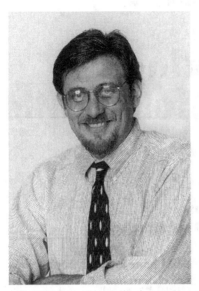

Ray Wycoff

Adam's driveway, Adam said, "Since Jeanne is out of town, why don't you have dinner with Susan and me?"

Ray shook his head. "Thanks anyway, I've got some work to do."

"It's no trouble, and work or no work, you've got to eat. Besides, I'd like to hear more about not being able to do your job."

There was a note on the kitchen table:

> Adam:
> Gone to office to finish up a document for a closing we have tomorrow a.m. Back about 8:30. Will bring pizza.
> Love you, Susan

Adam held the note up and announced: "Susan's at the real estate office. She'll be home in an hour or so with some mouth-watering cuisine from Italy. Perfect!"

The two men sat in canvas garden chairs on the back porch. Adam filled two glasses with iced water and raised his glass to gesture a toast, and Ray followed suit. "To solving problems!" Ray smiled.

Adam declared, "OK, let's have at it. What's the problem?"

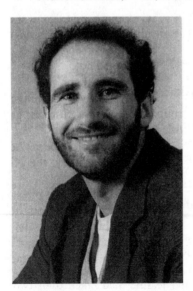

Adam Solomon

Ray paused a moment and then responded with a question of his own, "What would you do if you had information about a conspiracy in state government, information that you were able to determine was valid, and you were about to print it, only to have the governor inform you that you couldn't run it in the *Sentinel-Dispatch* or give it to anyone else?"

"Well, I'd remind Governor Baker that we have this little document called the Constitution, which has these amendments called the Bill of Rights. Then I'd direct his attention to numero uno, and then, after those courtesies, I'd print it!"

"Why would you print it?"

"You know very well why: In a democratic society, people have a right to

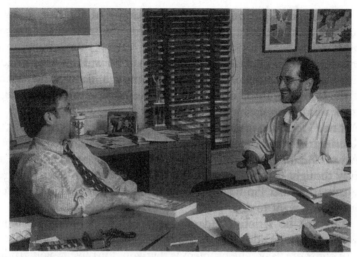

Ray Wycoff and Adam Solomon

know what is going on and, at the same time, the press has a moral obligation to inform the public of what's going on—hence the expression 'free press.' But I don't have to tell you that. What does all of this have to do with a director of public health who thinks he and his co-workers can't do their jobs?"

"Well, we are coming to the point where my colleagues and I are being told that we can't, metaphorically speaking, print the public health truth."

"Tell me more."

"We are being told in no uncertain terms that if we act on what we know to be the truth, what science tells us is the truth, our funds will be cut and our jobs will be at risk. We're stymied and we have no health 'bill of rights' to back us up."

Adam smiled. "That's a bit dramatic, isn't it? Besides, you folks are doing a lot—how about that Kids First campaign our paper helped you promote two years ago? Within a year, immunization coverage in Hillsdale reached its highest rate in history. Incidentally, I figure you guys couldn't buy the kind of coverage we gave you."

"Okay, point well taken, but there are still very important areas where we are simply being told 'hands off.' "

"By the governor?"

"Of course not."

"By whom, then?"

"Policymakers who themselves have been pressured by special-interest groups because those interest groups perceive our initiatives to be at odds with their special interests!"

With a hint of sarcasm, Adam interrupted, "We wouldn't be referring to the tobacco industry, the NRA, or the housing folks opposed to lead clean-up, would we?"

"Yes, we would. The pressure is all over the place. Last month I was at a meeting of epidemiologists from the military. They told me that a proposal to prohibit cigarette sales on military bases had been put forth and approved by the Department of Defense. They discovered later that the proposal had been tabled after members of Congress from certain tobacco-growing states had threatened to cut appropriations for base PXs. That's the kind of thing I'm talking about."

Adam grinned and stretched his arms upward. "Ah, sweet politics."

"It's not very funny to me, my friend."

Adam's smile disappeared. "From where I sit, public health is, by definition, political. And until you and your colleagues acknowledge that reality, and figure out how to operate within it, I suspect you'll probably continue to feel the way you do."

"Acknowledge it? Hell, we live it! Besides, there are very specific laws that prohibit public employees from lobbying for their causes."

"Au contraire, Ray. The problem is that you don't live it, you grudgingly tolerate it! I hear you saying that you are a recipient of the effects of being in a political arena; you're a victim. Frankly, I think that people outside your circle of colleagues will find that sounding a little like whining. If you want to avoid political victimization and the feeling of paralysis that inevitably accompanies it, then you have to become a player."

Ray stood up and strolled out onto the lawn behind the porch. Adam got up and followed him, fearing that he had gone too far and offended his friend. "Hey, I didn't mean to come on so strong."

"Actually, that's not what I was thinking at all. I suppose I do sound a bit whiny. Keep going."

"What I mean by becoming a player is to think and act proactively. To do that, you need a strategy to let people know who you are, what you do, and why it's important. And *you* can't be the only one doing the talking, Ray. You need others to get in the game, too. Real people who benefit from these programs and organizations besides the health department who think it's important and will be strong advocates. In my business, newspaper stories about health or social issues are more compelling when you can link them to a human face, an authentic voice, or a community outcry. Maybe I'm being naive, but I think the same formula works if you're trying to sell your story to policymakers or other decision leaders."

Ray couldn't mask his sarcasm in responding. "When you say 'sell your story,' it sounds like you want us to advertise!"

"Sounds as if you equate advertising with prostitution!"

Ray was silent.

Adam continued, "Tell me, do you really think the intent of advertising is that much different from the intent of what you call education and promotion?"

Ray got the point. "We're health people; we're not trained to go around telling people how good we are."

Adam interrupted, "Well, maybe you should be!"

"Look, we're so damn busy just keeping our heads above water, we don't have time to toot our own horns, even if we were of a mind to do so."

Adam paused and said, "It's not just about tooting your own horn, Ray. In fact, it's less about self-promotion than it is about building and making the strongest possible case for your cause. Find allies. Find beneficiaries. Gather evidence. Anticipate objections and be ready to address them. And most of all, pull these pieces together in a coordinated way that shows a community commitment to the problem. If you aren't willing to do that for something you really believe in, why would you expect that others who have much less invested in it than you would do the same? And frankly, that 'tooting your own horn' remark reflects an attitude that may be a big part of the problem."

"How so?" Ray asked.

"Would you agree that people in any community will speak out and support the institutions they value if those same institutions were somehow threatened?"

Ray nodded in agreement. Sounding like a trial lawyer, Adam continued, "Would you also agree that, currently, the public's general understanding of and appreciation for public health services is probably minimal?"

"Probably."

Adam looked at Ray and slowly enunciated, "That's . . . the . . . point!" pointing at his friend to emphasize each word. "How can you expect the people of Hillsdale to be supportive, especially in the face of political pressure and opposition from special interests, if they don't know what you do and why it is in their best interest for you to have their support to keep doing it? Incidentally, you need to understand that our paper does not, de facto, have a responsibility to promote public health! If you created a strategy to bring the merits of public health to the court of public opinion, two things would happen and they are both good."

"I assume that you will elaborate on those two things?" Ray asked knowingly.

"Of course. First, you would educate the community and probably make friends for public health that you wouldn't make otherwise. And second, that constant flow of information would serve to minimize the sensational effect that adversarial special-interest groups rely on."

Adam's reference to "making friends" triggered memories for Ray. "The mention of 'friends' of public health reminds me of an experience I had in my first year as health officer for the Greene County Health Department in Illinois."

"I have a nose for stories, and I sense one coming on."

"Can you tolerate it?" Ray asked.

"Only if it has a good title."

Ray thought for a moment and then said, "Let's call it 'Making Friends the Hard Way'!" He described how his health department had received a planning grant to put together an injury-prevention project proposal for a target area in the county. The proposal made good use of existing county-based data and highlighted the fact that his health department had established a strong collaboration with key county agencies, including the department of roads and transportation, emergency medical services, and the county sheriff's department. Ray had been adamant about his desire to secure the cooperation of other agencies. The planning team developed an impressive proposal that focused on reducing auto-related injuries among teenagers.

Ray explained that the week the proposal was due for submission to the state capital, he was asked to give a luncheon address at the Greene County Rotary Club meeting. He recalled how he had prepared his remarks to make the point that contemporary health problems are complex and not likely to be resolved without extensive cooperation among many sectors of the community. To illustrate his point, Ray used the proposed injury-prevention program as a concrete illustration of action under way. With great enthusiasm, he described key elements of the program and showed a county map, highlighting the high-priority target areas.

The discussion period following his presentation was a disaster. It began when a coach from the high school indicated that he strongly favored an injury-prevention program, but that this occasion was the first time he had heard about it; he asked if it was too late to involve the school system, implying that the school district had been left out. Ray knew that there had been a school representative on the planning committee, but she had left the area at the end of the school year to take a new position in another part of the state. Most of the planning had taken place in the summer and no replacement had been found.

"Once the coach had spoken, I felt like I was the bait for a shark's feeding frenzy."

Adam was now fully engaged. "What happened?"

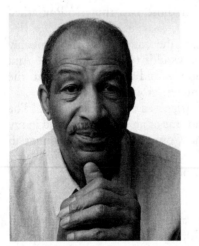

Reverend Carver

Ray described how Reverend Carver, the next speaker, stood up and politely but firmly questioned the department's priorities. The reverend observed that the main target area for the program was adjacent to low-income neighborhoods with serious housing, employment, and basic health needs.

Ray stretched his right arm up about a foot over his own head, and looked at Adam. "Reverend Carver is an imposing figure—a big man with a soft voice. As I recall, he said something like 'Once again we see another example of the government deciding what the people want and need. The residents of the West End, which my church serves, are poor. Like all poor people, they bear a greater burden of illness than the rest of the community. Wouldn't it make more sense to spend your resources on the real causes of poor health—things like inferior housing and no jobs?'"

Ray had tried to explain that he understood the reverend's point, but that the money for the program was earmarked for injury prevention and could not be used for matters like housing and unemployment.

· "The reverend politely heard my response, then rhetorically asked, 'Why not?' and sat down. I had no retort."

"And then you made friends?" Adam asked.

"No, then the floodgates opened. Others expressed their concerns. The most notable was the director of Mothers Against Drunk Driving, who indicated that while she was pleased to hear that the health department was getting involved with this important problem, she was disappointed to have to hear about it in a public meeting at a point when the program was apparently a fait accompli. She expressed disappointment at being ignored in the planning effort, even though MADD had been successful in bringing stiffer law enforcement and penalties for driving under the influence of alcohol."

Ray paused, "I was stunned. If I had been talking about the merits of sex education as a means to prevent the spread of HIV/AIDS, or even water fluoridation, I would have anticipated some flack. But injury prevention?"

"Fair enough," Adam said, "but surely you've been in their situation and know what that feels like, right?"

Ray thought for a minute. "Actually, I'm in a similar situation right now. How ironic that I never put the two together. Remember the story you guys ran a few months back about the new statewide initiative on bioterrorism preparedness? Well, it turns out that it's no simple task to coordinate the participation and roles of all the key players. You've got first responders like police and fire departments, medical and nursing staff, infectious disease experts, and civic and public health leaders, and all of them have their own responsibilities and priorities. And education of the public is another challenge altogether. I'm on the state committee, and I keep suggesting that this is exactly the sort of thing that our public health educators are trained to do, and that we should get them involved in a major way. But so far, no one seems to be listening."

"Okay, get back to the original story now," said Adam. "Where does the making friends part come in?"

"Well," Ray said, "the next day, I made an appointment to meet with Reverend Carver out in the West End. I was motivated partly because I wanted to mend fences, but also I wanted to learn what went wrong. I discovered two things. First, even though I'd lived in Greene County for many years, I realized there were areas I didn't really know at all. Second, and this is related to the first point, it struck me that when you cut through all the theories and words, good communication comes down to having respect for people's views. It means seeking out those you may not ordinarily encounter and listening carefully to their, ideas, concerns, and priorities."

By urging him to be more aggressive about taking the story of public health to the public, Adam had helped Ray see the connection between increasing community awareness about the value of public health and grass-roots participation. Adam also made Ray realize that community participation in public health wouldn't occur unless he made it a priority to meet with people and listen to them.

Adam thought for a moment and then spoke. "You know, most leaders and managers are struggling with change just like you are. For most of us, the social context in which we do our work has changed, but we haven't. It's as if we're experienced players in a game where the rules have been radically changed!"

"And those changes for me are political?"

"It seems that way to me. But when you say 'political,' it's as if you're saying 'corrupt.' Also, earlier you said that as a public employee you couldn't lobby. That tells me that you believe you have to lobby or buy favors to be a player in the political arena."

"A lot of people feel that way."

"Wait here a minute." Adam moved briskly into the house. A few moments later he returned, carrying a huge dictionary and a thin red paperback. He put the small book down and began to flip through the pages of the dictionary. "Remember, I'm a newspaper guy and words are my business, and 'political' is a big word. Ah, here we are."

Adam handed Ray the dictionary and pointed to a spot on the page. "Scan these definitions, starting with the word 'politic,' through to 'politicize.'"

Ray read to himself and then said, "Here it is. 'Crafty,' 'unscrupulous,' . . . Here's a good one, listen to this: '. . . scheming, opportunism, etc., as opposed to a statesman, which suggests able, far-seeing, principled conduct.' I love the 'etc.' part! I rest my case." Ray felt like a poker player who had just successfully drawn to an inside straight.

Adam grinned. "By resting your case, my friend, you have helped me make mine! One of the curious things about the words 'politics,' 'political,' and 'politician' is that they have two sides: a negative side, which you chose to highlight, and a positive side, which you chose to ignore. Allow me." Adam took the dictionary from Ray's hands, studied the page for a moment, and said, "For example, you didn't mention such things as 'having practical wisdom,' 'prudent,' 'diplomatic,' 'concerned with government'—or how about this under political liberty: 'the right to participate in determining the form, choosing the officials, making the laws, and carrying on the function of one's government'?"

Adam handed the dictionary to Ray and picked up the paperback. "There's a phrase in here I have always liked. Here it is." He cleared his throat to dramatize his reading, ". . . the term 'political' is not inherently negative; it comes from the Greek notion of *polis* and refers to a place where governance was achieved through dialogue and advocacy, and it is balanced by study and inquiry."[1] He looked at Ray, "A bit idealistic, perhaps, but nice, don't you think?"

Ray thought to himself, A full house beats a straight! "Yes, very nice. Point well taken."

Adam went on, "For centuries, playwrights and novelists have dramatized humanity's struggle with the forces of good and evil, and the political arena has been one of the prime settings for playing out that struggle. Rather than being inherently good or bad, politics is just real. One can be a greedy and corrupt player, or one who plays with principles and dignity. For you public health folks, the choice isn't whether to play, but how you're going to balance the struggle in favor of integrity."

At that moment, Susan pulled back the sliding door to the back porch and announced, "Anyone for a little pizza with fresh eggplant, mushrooms, tomatoes, black olives, and pepperoni?"

Case Analysis

How many community health workers, with the heartfelt intentions of a Don Quixote, have had their dreams dashed by the churning blades of political windmills? The "Court of Public Opinion" case story calls our attention to the reality that social and political forces do indeed influence the ability of practitioners to plan and deliver effective community health promotion programs. We are reminded of three points: (1) public health practice is inseparably tied to the political workings of the community it seeks to serve; (2) it is unreasonable to think that effective public health practice can be implemented and sustained if it is invisible to the general public and community decision makers; and (3) failure to seek and respect the counsel of citizens reflects a flaw in both the ethics and the application of public health programs.

The remainder of this chapter is divided into two sections offering ideas and actions that will help health promotion practitioners work more effectively within the political realities of the communities they serve. In the first section, "Participation," we review the scientific and ethical rationale for actively seeking citizen participation, and recommend some practical approaches for securing that participation. In the second section, "Building Political and Public Support," we outline a strategic approach to increase awareness about the purpose and value of public health. This section also describes tactics for reaching various audiences.

PARTICIPATION

The word *participate* means to share or take part with others in some activity or enterprise. With regard to health promotion activities and programs, we think it is useful to think of community participation as having two complementary dimensions. One refers to the participation of multiple organizations in the planning and delivery of health promotion programs; the other refers to circumstances where community members are seen not merely as recipients of a program, but rather as active participants in shaping and implementing that program.

In this section, we emphasize the latter point. In doing so, however, we offer practitioners two cautions:

Caution 1. Do not minimize the importance of reaching out and establishing partnerships with organizations and groups whose participation can enhance your efforts to improve the health of the community you serve. It goes without saying that a local health department would be in for a rude awakening if it tried to launch a breast cancer screening program without coordinating with its local volunteer cancer agency and local physicians.

Caution 2. We all understand that heavy-handed, expert-only decision making in communities is a formula for disaster. At the same time, the need to enhance citizen participation should not be mistaken as a call for practitioners to apologize for their training and experience and to abdicate their professional skills and knowledge. The enemies of true participation are those who create divisiveness by their relentless pursuit of the "right" answer or the "right" way. Convergence of differing points will result from a combination of common courtesy, listening, and a genuine desire to achieve something better. Our best advice is simple: Don't use "listening" as a tactic and then "lay on" your expertise. Listen to learn, and then be honest in your own response.

Recall Ray Wycoff's experience in Greene County. The planning team had reasonable representation from multiple organizations, and it did come up with a scientifically sound program idea. But even though the group's interorganizational and scientific ducks seemed to be in order, its failure to take into account the values and interests of the individuals it was trying to reach led to difficulties.

WHY IS PARTICIPATION IMPORTANT?

Consider the nature of the problems practitioners work on and the context in which they address them. Over the years, findings from epidemiologic and behavioral science research have given us a better understanding of the factors and circumstances that seem to shape and even predict the preventable problems you are likely to face in your community: heart disease, cancer, injuries, suicide, homicide, alcohol and drug abuse, teen pregnancy, age-related problems, HIV/AIDS, and so on. The factors and circumstances that explain the occurrence of these health problems are often expressed as a causal chain.

In theory, if you know the elements of the causal chain and can modify them, chances are that you can prevent the problem in question. But the term *causal chain* paints a deceptive picture of linear order. In reality, it is a very messy, convoluted chain! It is a mixture of biological, behavioral, environmental, political, and economic factors.

Furthermore, few if any of these factors are stable; not only will they vary in degree over time, but they will also vary from country to country, state to state, province to province, community to community, neighborhood to neighborhood, and so on. Given the inevitability that practitioners must address complex, moving targets, it is safe to say that programs and policies aimed at preventing such problems are not likely to be effective without the informed, active involvement of individuals, families, and local groups and institutions. This is especially true when one tries to undertake a public policy or legislative approach to health promotion or disease prevention.

No doubt many of us can identify with Ray Wycoff's experience in Greene County: the gnawing truth that we failed to engage people who should have been involved. Based on our experience, we believe that such failure is most often the result of an unintended error of omission, caused primarily by the practitioner's failure to keep sight of the principle of participation. Of all the concepts that help shape research and practice in community health promotion, none generates more consensus than the citizen dimension of community participation. The following frequently cited passage from the 1974 Alma-Ata Declaration captures not only the intent of the concept, but its relevance and ethic as well: ". . . people have the right and the duty to participate individually and collectively in the planning and implementing of their health care."[2]

A well-trained, talented, and experienced person is capable of solving problems and overcoming challenges that might baffle others who are less talented and less experienced. In many jobs, talented people can carry out their work with minimal or no involvement of those who receive their services. Examples include the expert plumber, microbiologist, auto mechanic, chemist, or tailor. Such is not the case for capable community health promotion practitioners. A key element of their competency is the capacity to engage community members and elicit their participation in all phases of their work: planning, implementation, and evaluation. This element of community participation must be an integral part of the practitioner's mental model.

In 1986, Lawrence Green introduced a set of propositions for the purpose of validating theories of participation.[3] We have modified these propositions and offer them up as a means to test your own mental model with respect to participation. As you read each of the propositions below, ask yourself, "To what extent is this statement consistent with my own beliefs?"

1. As the level of active—as opposed to passive—participation of people in the planning and implementation process increases, the probability of achieving health improvement goals will also increase.

2. Both active participation and consensus will increase as people are engaged, listened to, and informed about community health status and opportunities for health improvement.

3. As people receive feedback on the progress of programs and services they have had a hand in shaping, their trust and participation will increase.

Editorial squabbles aside, community health promotion practitioners who have difficulty acting on these propositions are likely to repeat the experiences Ray Wycoff had in Greene County.

When practitioners think about engaging the community, one of the first things to come to mind is the notion of a community coalition— a group of people representative of a community, coalesced by the shared interest to achieve a common vision. The success of that coalition is testimony to common sense: dictatorships aside, representative groups can accomplish what one person cannot.

Assembling a coalition or working group is one thing; managing and keeping that group on track is another. Even with the best of intentions, problems can arise that disrupt or even destroy the spirit of cooperative group process. If practitioners are sensitive and alert to these problems, the majority of problems can be prevented or at least minimized.

Following are examples of several problems that commonly come to the surface. We express these problems as symptoms and give examples of how those symptoms surface in day-to-day practice. We then offer examples of specific steps (tactics) that might be taken to address those symptoms or to prevent them from arising. As you read through the examples, keep in mind that healthy, productive coalitions are never free of conflict; problems and disagreements are inherent and often beneficial in a truly robust planning process. The challenge is to anticipate and prevent unnecessary problems and to manage disagreement and conflict.

Symptom 1: Members of organizations not included in the planning activities resist your planning process and proposals.

Example.   A group of physicians who have been working on breast cancer screening have not been consulted by your group as you develop plans for a more comprehensive cancer prevention and control program. As your group presents its plan for funding and support, the physician group gets word to key decision makers that the resources in question would be more efficiently spent on their existing mammography program. With such input from a reputable group, the decision makers are likely to put your request for support on hold until some clarification is achieved.

Tactic.   To minimize the chance of such opposition, place a priority (early on and throughout the planning process) on notifying and querying all parties and organizations that might have an interest or an investment in some aspect of the issue or problem you plan to address. This can be accomplished by taking the following action steps:

- Ask all persons involved in the initiation of the planning to identify organizations or individuals who may have an interest or stake in the issue at hand. Planning group members should be encouraged to make personal contact with those organizations or individuals to inform them of your intentions and to determine their level of interest.

- Develop written communications (newsletters, memos, electronic mail) and disseminate them through existing community channels.

- Develop and implement a policy to make formal announcements in public meetings or through mass-media channels. In all communications, include a request for inquiries and ideas.

Symptom 2: The coalition's business is disrupted by members of the group who argue about the direction that is being taken; competing agendas become problematic.

Example. A member of the planning group is adamant about moving as quickly as possible to implement a cervical cancer screening program for a low-income population because "the problem is evident." This person has expressed strong opposition to recommendations of the health department representative who has been urging the group to give priority to an epidemiologic analysis of women's health problems, which has not yet been done for the proposed target area. The conflict is a classic case of "it needs further study" versus "we need to act now."

Tactic. Because such spirited differences are commonplace, we encourage leaders to view such moments as opportunities for growth. Consider these actions:

- Early in the process of selecting members of the planning team, ask members to (1) declare the mission of their agency or organization or the bias they bring as an unaffiliated member, and (2) describe how the "vision" the planning group seeks is related to their mission or personal bias. Indicate to them what roles they will and will not be permitted to play.

- When conflict arises over vested interests, encourage the relevant parties to reexamine the vision and mission statements and use those as a means to return their discussion to common ground. In the example given here, the point should be made that both goals have merit. Help resolve the conflict by assisting in reframing the problem. Rather than debating the merits of program implementation versus data collection and analysis, the question should be, "How can we have useful data without depleting needed program resources and unduly delaying implementation?" Keep everyone focused on the vision.

Symptom 3: Participation in the coalition declines and becomes limited to a small group representing a narrow range of interest, often accompanied by reports of "burnout."

Example. There is high turnout and great enthusiasm during the first two planning meetings. Then, with each subsequent meeting, you notice a steady decline in attendance. A small core of participants maintains the burden. There is talk of burnout and attendance becomes sporadic. In retrospect, you found it easy to form the planning group but difficult to maintain it.

Tactic. Depending on the circumstances, it may take a year to complete the planning process. It is unrealistic to expect many people, who are already busy and committed to their day-to-day routines, to have the time and energy to stay with a long and demanding planning process. Following are strategic steps to increase planning efficiency and keep the time burden manageable for members of the planning team:

- In your first meeting, use clear, concise agendas designed to address the highest-priority issues. Indicate that few large-group meetings will occur; those that are held will be kept short.

- Distribute and manage the tasks. Planning group members have varied interests. Determine their special areas of interest and form small "task groups" based on those interests. Through the collective input of the planning group in early meetings, delineate specific activities for the respective task groups and determine when, in the course of the planning process, the product of their activity is due. This small task group approach will help maintain the integrity of the planning team by allowing members (1) to move in and out of the planning process as their expertise is needed, thus reducing the time burden, and (2) to focus on those issues most closely associated with their priorities and expertise.

- Develop a Gantt chart, showing which tasks are due at what time; make this chart available to all members of the planning team.

- To keep all members informed of key issues and progress, publish a planning team communiqué or newsletter at regular intervals.

Symptom 4: Actions and intentions of the planning group or coalition are misrepresented either in the media or in public discussions.

Example. As a result of your planning process, comprehensive school health education has emerged as a key element for a proposed community health promotion program. Your group is surprised when an article appears in the newspaper revealing that a group of "concerned citizens" is alarmed because your proposal for comprehensive school health is really a cover for a liberal "sex education" program. The article is followed by TV news coverage, and various agency cosponsors involved in the planning receive queries. Many people start asking, "What's going on?"

Tactic. Early in the planning process, set aside specific time to anticipate efforts by those who would try to misrepresent your intentions. Continually ask questions like "Who needs to be informed of our activities?" and "How might a given activity be misinterpreted?" Develop a strategy to keep all members of the planning team (and the key decision makers in the organizations they represent) routinely informed. Any one, or a combination, of the following techniques, will promote such awareness: (1) a regular newsletter, (2) periodic briefing or update sessions, or (3) special memos alerting relevant parties of key or potentially controversial issues. Establish a liaison for dealing with representatives from the local print and electronic media (it is ideal to have a media person on the planning team). News items on key issues and outcomes of the planning process not only increase the visibility of the proposed program and heighten public awareness, but also serve to reinforce the significance of the planning process in the eyes of the planning team members.

Symptom 5: "Plain folks" don't seem to be interested in participating.

Example. At your first coalition meeting, you look around the table and see that everyone in attendance is a paid staff member from one of the major health-related organizations or agencies in town. Moreover, you already know most of them on a first-name basis. Despite all your talk about community involvement and participation, this group looks like the usual suspects.

Be careful not to romanticize the principle of community participation. The idealist in you wants to believe that community residents long for the opportunity to participate in the planning of health promotion programs and, if only given the chance, will drop everything and participate with the same level of commitment as those who are paid to do so as professionals. The pragmatist in you realizes that many people have no interest in participating. Among those who do, most tend to get involved with issues and problems they perceive as serious and relevant in their own lives.

The following tactics are designed to help gain the involvement of a wider range of community residents, so that the ideals of citizen participation can be pursued without ignoring the challenges that exist in reality.

Tactic 1. Gather information about the population, or populations, your program is supposed to serve. Where do you start? Suppose you are traveling across the country and your car breaks down on a Friday night in an area you know nothing about. You're told your car can't be fixed until Monday afternoon or Tuesday. In addition to "asking around," one of the fastest ways to find out something about the place you're in is to scan the local newspaper. Whether it is a monthly, weekly, or daily publication, it will give you a good deal of insight about the place through news features, announcements, a calendar of events, and advertisements.

The extent to which one learns about a community is largely dependent upon the desire to do so, as we saw when Ray Wycoff drove out to see Reverend Carver. The point here is that practitioners need to drive out to meet their Reverend Carvers before being shamed into doing so. As a health promotion practitioner, you may have access to existing records and data sources. If so, you should use them to create a demographic and epidemiologic profile that will help you sharpen your picture of the people and their community.

Tactic 2. In some instances, especially where racial, cultural, ethnic, and/or socioeconomic diversity come into play, gaining the trust and participation of community members can pose unique challenges. Sadly, the experience with community health promotion programs in many minority or underserved communities has been one of promises not kept and disappointment. Consequently, as Ron Braithwaite and his colleagues have observed, in some instances you should prepare for a "period of suspicion."[4] Building relationships and partnerships with indigenous leaders or "gatekeepers" (neighborhood leaders, local service providers, business owners, clergy, youth workers, teachers, senior citizen workers) can help not only in gaining entrée to the community, but also in building and sustaining productive participation among residents and community organizations. Patience and persistence are also needed. Avoid the mistake of underestimating how much time and effort will be needed to establish community rapport and trust.

Tactic 3. Contact local institutions. Kretzman and McKnight found that local libraries serve as a central meeting place for many community organizations.[5] The librarian can give you information on groups that meet there, and sometimes libraries keep a self-published directory of local organizations. Besides health-related groups, local organizations to contact might include churches, parks and recreation departments, schools, law enforcement agencies, art or cultural centers, and business associations.

Tactic 4. Apply the awareness-raising tactics spelled out earlier in this chapter to let people in the community know about opportunities for participating in health promotion programs and activities.

Tactic 5. Use incentives and recognition as a part of your efforts to recruit and sustain participation.

Tactic 6. Invite community members to participate in a seminar that highlights key health issues and to share their ideas about those issues. Use such gatherings and events to survey attendees and assess their willingness and interest in participating; identify the skills they have and what roles they might be willing to play as part of an emerging health initiative.

A serious commitment to engaging community members in your work is a direct reflection of respect: a deferential regard to a fellow citizen, the acknowledgment of worth. The following is an excerpt from an essay written by Kentucky essayist Wendell Berry.[6] In this piece, Berry describes meeting a fellow Kentuckian and discovering that they have something in common. We share this story because it captures the spirit and power of community respect.

> "I've heard of Middletown," I said. "It was the home of my father's great friend, John W. Jones."
>
> "Well, John W. Jones was my uncle."
>
> I told him then of my father's and my own respect for Mr. Jones.

"I want to tell you a story about Uncle John," he said. And he told me this:

When his Uncle John was president of the bank in North Middletown, his policy was to give a loan to any graduate of the North Middletown High School who wanted to go to college and needed the money. This practice caused great consternation to the bank examiners who came and found those unsecured loans on the books and no justification for them except Mr. Jones's conviction that it was right to make them.

As it turned out, it was right in more than principle, for in the many years that Mr. Jones was president of the bank, making those "unsound loans," all of the loans were repaid; he never lost a dime on a one of them.

I do not mean to raise here the question of the invariable goodness of a college education, which I doubt. My point in telling this story is that Mr. Jones was acting from a kind of knowledge, inestimably valuable and probably indispensable, that comes out of common culture and that cannot be taught as a part of the formal curriculum of a school ... what he knew—and this involved his knowledge of himself, his tradition, his community, and everybody in it—was that trust, in the circumstances then present, could beget trustworthiness. This is the kind of knowledge, obviously, that is fundamental to the possibility of community life and to certain good possibilities in the character of people.

Applying these six tactics has never been more important than it is right now. In *Healthy People 2010,* one of the two overarching health promotion goals for the United States is to eliminate health disparities that exist between different populations. Achieving this goal will require an intensified focus on increasing participation among members of those groups that suffer from such disparities. By engaging populations in meaningful ways in planning, designing, implementing, and evaluating health promotion programs and policies, health promotion practitioners can better understand not only the causes of disparities, but also potential solutions.

BUILDING POLITICAL AND PUBLIC SUPPORT

A second lesson from this chapter's case story is that political and public support for health promotion and public health can be stimulated if efforts are made to do so. Because the benefits of such support can be substantial, we provide in this section specific strategies and tactics to help health promotion practitioners participate in this important activity.

From Geoffrey Rose's insightful book, *The Strategy of Preventive Medicine,* we find this wisdom:

Political decisions are for the politicians. Their agenda is complex, and mostly hidden from public scrutiny. This is unfortunate, because often the public would give higher priority to health than those who formulate political policies. Anything that stimulates more public information and debate on health issues is good, not just because it may lead to healthier choices, but also because it earns a high place for health issues on the political agenda. In the long run, this is probably the most important achievement of health education.[7]

Professor Rose would have been a good reference to reinforce Adam Solomon's "prompting" of Ray Wycoff. Rose's insight also was empirically confirmed in a 1994 study conducted by Macro International and funded by the CDC.[8] A part of the study sought to ascertain the extent to which the American public understands the goals, purpose, and value of public health. Findings from the study suggested that the average citizen has little or no understanding of either the scope or the significance of public health. For example, when citizens were asked, "What comes to mind when I mention public health?" typical responses included:

- "Restaurant inspections"
- "Free immunizations"
- "Doctors for the poor"
- "The ugly pink building downtown"

More specifically, the study identified several misperceptions and attitudes that, if left unaddressed, would tend to undermine efforts to create support for public health. These included the following:

- Limited awareness of public health's scope and significance
- Strong and exclusive association of public health and health departments as one and the same, delivering services for the poor
- Misplaced confidence that public health functions can be and will be performed by others (the National Guard, in one example!)
- Skepticism and misinterpretation of data on public health priorities and benefits, creating an "information vacuum" on public health issues
- Conflicting values between public health positions on some issues and those of churches and community groups
- Concern about the intrusiveness of lifestyle messages
- Resentment of public health's regulatory role
- Generic antigovernment sentiment; a feeling that public health is yet another waste of tax dollars

Although these responses confirm why public health is often referred to as a "silent miracle," analysis of the focus-group interviews also yielded several encouraging themes:

- Appreciation for public health's role can be readily stimulated—that is, public health functions that are taken for granted (like clean water, environmental protection, and immunizations) are appreciated once an effort has been made to point out the benefits.

- If informed, people will acknowledge that they benefit from public health, even if they never set foot in the health department.

- Like politics, public health is local. Therefore, when looking for a compelling example of the benefits and value of good public health, look to your own backyard first for those examples.

- Even though they may be resistant to the regulatory roles of public health, people understand that public health regulations are indeed protective and reassuring.

The information about the specific misperceptions some people hold, combined with the insight that there are real ways to address those misperceptions, led to the formulation of some key "message concepts" that were deemed most likely to enlighten community members about the importance and value of public health:

Public health works. Such messages highlight public health's many accomplishments and counter negative views of wasteful, ineffective bureaucracies. Public health is cost-effective.

Prevention works and is a good investment. Prevention services encompass everything from immunization to health education to restaurant inspections that prevent food-borne pathogens. When we invest, we want two things: profit and value. An investment in health improvement that emphasizes prevention will achieve both goals. Profit will manifest itself in greater productivity and improved quality of life. Value will be created because for a large portion of contemporary health problems, effective prevention yields positive health outcomes at a lower cost than does awaiting treatment.[9]

Public health protects you and your family. This concept highlights the fact that public health offers confidence in daily life—that food and water are safe, that new diseases will be detected and countered, that accurate information on health and environmental issues will be available. Thus public health is for everyone, not just the poor and disadvantaged who are in need of special medical services.

Only public health has a mandate to address the health of everyone in your community. This message reinforces the protective aspect of public health and applies to entire communities as well as to individuals and families. This message concept also captures the unique role of public health in monitoring health status and documenting progress in combating diseases, injuries, and disabilities.

Public health is always there. During disasters, the public turns to public health. Public health's emergency-response role, while sporadic and not applicable in every community, is reassuring and highlights many of public health's otherwise invisible features: rapid response, accurate information, setting priorities, looking out for the community's interests, and preventing disease, to name a few.

Public health is indispensable. Without public health, our quality of life would be palpably worse. We would lose confidence in the safety of our environment and would feel more vulnerable to preventable diseases. We would not know as much about the health status of our communities, nor would we have the information and expertise to address health problems. Without public health, the costs of treating medical conditions, which already account for most of our health care expenditures, would increase even faster.

These message concepts, when applied as a part of a health communications and media advocacy strategy, increase the likelihood of getting public health on your community's map.

A Cautionary Note.   Attitudes and perceptions about public health and health promotion will vary across communities. Therefore, before undertaking any of the tactical options described, practitioners should think strategically and follow the same careful diagnostic procedures that have been emphasized throughout this book.

Getting the public health message out is complicated by the reality that, to be effective, you need to reach several audiences with your message.[10] To better manage that complexity, we have found the following process to be helpful. First, delineate all of the possible audiences you need to reach. Next, to help you think strategically, choose one of those audiences. Once you have determined your target audience, answers to the following questions will generate the information that will keep you on track:

How does the target audience perceive public health?

Given the audience's perceptions, what ideas about benefits of public health do I want to communicate?

What objective do I want to achieve?

What materials do I need to achieve the objective?

Repeat the same process for all of the target audiences you plan to reach. For example, suppose that one of your key audiences consists of state legislators or county commissioners. By interviewing some of them and/or obtaining information from their voting records, media interviews, or other published statements, you could develop answers to these four questions. A number of possible answers are provided in Table 3.1.

TABLE 3.1 Communications Planning Matrix

Audience-Specific Problems/Misconceptions	Communication Objective(s)	Concepts/Materials	Benefits Perceived By Audience
Legislators/County Commissioners • Limited awareness of public health's scope • Antibureaucratic, antiregulatory sentiment • Skepticism toward cost-benefit and other data • "Values" conflict	• Increase sense of public health's relevance and importance • Increase appreciation for positive regulatory role (clean water, safe food), cost-effectiveness, and efficiency of public health services • Highlight "neutral" activities that benefit the community at large	• Responsibility for the community's health ("Day in the Life"*) • Public health works: cost-benefit tied to legislator's interests and a human story • "Day in the Life" and other local examples ("Did you know that . . . ?") • Health status report card	• Public health affects me and my constituents, not just "them" • Public health is a worthwhile investment • It's more than condoms in schools, needle exchange, etc. Life would be more dangerous, unpleasant, uncertain, etc. without these services
Boards of Health • Where public health fits in the spectrum of community health services	• Support public health with media, legislators, public	• Cost-benefit information on prevention activities • Health status report	• Public health is a major contributor to our community's health
Managed Care Organizations • Turf issues: Who will be responsible for which services under health reform? • With universal coverage, public health may not be needed	• Partnership with public health to support prevention goals and share data relevant to community health	• Cost-benefit information • Health status report • Unique public health contributions/expertise (e.g., outreach)	• Public health is a key partner for our organization • Public health plays an essential role beyond service provision

(continued)

TABLE 3.1 *Continued*

Audience-Specific Problems/Misconceptions	Communication Objective(s)	Concepts/Materials	Benefits Perceived By Audience
Media			
• Perception that public health topics are boring to readers/viewers/listeners • Limited awareness • Public health is clinics for the poor • Public health may no longer be necessary after health care reform	• Increase knowledge and understanding of essential services • Increase awareness of public health's contributions to community health • Increase appreciation for cost-benefit of investment in public health	• "Day in the Life" • Scenarios: what would happen in our community without public health? • Health status report card • "Investigative" angle: investments in prenatal care, TB outreach, or AIDS counseling saved X, but funding is being cut	• Public health is interesting and relevant to me and to my readers or viewers • Public health has a human angle • A strong public health system is essential; the media have a role in covering this topic and reminding legislators of its importance
General Public			
• Limited awareness • Public health is only for poor people; it does not apply to me • Public health is a wasteful bureaucracy • Public health is trying to tell me how to live my life	• Increase awareness of scope and benefits • Show public health's efficiency in its own right, and compared to other expenditures • Demonstrate benefits of public health lifestyle messages	• "Day in the Life" • Public health works • Spokespersons for public health — "What it does for me" • Scenarios—without public health, what would happen?	• Public health protects and serves me, whether I use the health department or not • My family and I need a strong public health system

* "A Day in the Life of Public Health" is a one-page narrative describing the many ways a typical middle-class person benefits from public health — without ever setting foot in the health department. It was developed in 1993 by the Colorado Department of Health.

HEIGHTENING PUBLIC AWARENESS: STRATEGIC THINKING

Those responsible for planning and implementing public-awareness campaigns will find the following six strategies, and the specific tactics to carry them out, helpful.

Strategy 1: Develop and Nurture Relationships with Management and Editorial Staff in the Local Media

Tactic 1.1. Invite reporters, key management, and editorial staff from local media to brown-bag lunches, workshops, and meetings that highlight late-breaking public health issues, key programs, or progress reports.

Tactic 1.2. Take the time to meet with representatives from the media in your community and determine what motivates them and what specific needs they have that public health practitioners can help fulfill. This action responds to the point that Adam Solomon made in the case story: The media do not have a de facto responsibility to promote public health.

Tactic 1.3. Promote the development of designated health department staff members as expert consultants to contact when the media want to report on a local public health crisis (e.g., an infectious disease outbreak) or to localize a national public health story.

Tactic 1.4. Help practitioners portray public health as a system by encouraging them to show how various public health activities are interdependent. For example, if a health department is asked to describe its immunization program, public health workers can show continuity by explaining (1) how assessment activities are essential for monitoring trends in the cases of measles in the community; (2) how policies based on disease surveillance ensure timely vaccination of children; (3) how the health department ensures the availability of immunization services and vaccines; and (4) how high rates of immunization coverage not only prevent disease but also increase the likelihood that children will be able to experience the social and educational benefits of attending school.

Strategy 2: Implement a Training Program to Enhance Practitioners' Skills in Media Advocacy

Tactic 2.1. Meet with the leader of your local health department to get support to create and manage a series of seminars designed to orient community public health leaders, practitioners, and public health advocates in the process of media advocacy.[11]

Tactic 2.2. Develop the curriculum with a primary emphasis on (1) reframing public debate to increase public support for more effective policy-level approaches to public health problems and (2) fostering the media's role in setting the public agenda and stimulating public discussion around public health issues.

Tactic 2.3. Develop practical skill-building sessions where participants can learn and practice how to (1) apply "social math," (2) "frame" issues, and (3) gain access to media outlets.

Strategy 3: With Your Community or Service Area, Participate in National Public Health Week to Highlight the Significance of Public Health to the Health of Your Community, State, and Nation

(Note: The first week in April has been designated as National Public Health Week in the United States. By participating in a public health week in your community, especially one that coincides with a state or national event, you increase your opportunities for positive exposure and promotion of public health and prevention.)

Tactic 3.1. Work with public health leaders in your community to encourage local government officials to formally declare that one week per year be designated as Public Health Week. If possible, the date should coincide with national efforts to gain from those larger promotional and media benefits.

Tactic 3.2. Establish a Public Health Week consortium of organizations that support the principles of public health. Such a consortium might include local print and electronic media, volunteer organizations, hospitals, managed-care groups, insurance companies, public schools, libraries, service clubs, athletic and sports organizations, and businesses.

Tactic 3.3. Practitioners in the United States should contact the National Association of County and City Health Officials (NACCHO) and request their Health Day Starter Kit. This kit contains sample governmental proclamations, message ideas, and promotional materials, along with tips on activities to highlight during the week.

Strategy 4: Make the Public Aware That Public Health Services Are Essential

Tactic 4.1. Have an inspector take local media or community representatives along on inspections of child-care centers to illustrate the role of essential services in maintaining safe facilities for the community's children.

Strategy 5: Make Data Understandable and More Relevant

Tactic 5.1. Meet with the health reporter for your local newspaper and offer to generate analyses of health data that he or she can put into a periodic "Health Factoid" feature (as appears in *USA Today*, for example).

Tactic 5.2. Hold a data-sharing seminar with other organizations, where you indicate that your data may be used by their organizations to develop programs and plan activities.

Tactic 5.3. Be prepared to take advantage of opportunities to discuss local or state data when a national survey on a health issue hits the press.

Tactic 5.4. Publish a comprehensive report card on the health status of the community that includes specific indicators, essential services conducted to derive those data, the specific division of the health department responsible for those indicators, and any other services or programs that address those indicators.

Tactic 5.5. A story reporting a severe health problem or disease outbreak in another area or county can provide a timely opportunity to educate citizens in your community about the essential protective services that your health department provides. For example, if an outbreak of a waterborne disease is reported in a nearby city, your local media may find it newsworthy to publish a story asking "How Safe Are We Here?" If justified, such a story could be a key vehicle to inform the public about why their support for a public health infrastructure has value.

Strategy 6: Reach the Decision Makers

Tactic 6.1. With fellow public health advocates, adopt a decision maker![12] Make contact and establish a relationship. If the decision maker in question is a legislator, your best chances to make contact are likely to be through a staff member. Listen to the decision maker and pay attention. Find out what he or she knows and believes about health. Become the decision maker's resource and expert on public health issues. If such a relationship is viewed as too political, work with other advocates to fill such a role: university professors, graduate students, retired former health workers, and members of volunteer health organizations.

Tactic 6.2. Sponsor conferences or seminars on public and community health for decision makers and practitioners. Such conferences create opportunities for interaction between public health practitioners and state legislators. Meals and social gatherings at these events provide an informal setting for learning and exchanging ideas.

Tactic 6.3. Examine the evaluations you have conducted of your health promotion and disease prevention programs. Where data permit, use cost-effectiveness and cost-benefit analysis to show program value and comparative savings. When using data, translate the information into messages and images that make it clear that real people are behind the numbers.

SUMMARY

"Rich together, poor if separated" (Laos); "one finger cannot lift a pebble" (Iran); "united we stand, divided we fall" (United States). These memorable phrases and countless others like them suggest that, regardless of cultural differences, the idea of people forming alliances to accomplish valued outcomes, including health, is universal.

The concept of "community" has long been a fundamental component in the design and implementation of health and social programs. In 1923,

C. E. A. Winslow offered this definition of public health (the italics are ours):

> the science and art of preventing disease, prolonging life, and pro-
> moting health and well-being *through organized community efforts*
> for the sanitation of the environment, the control of communica-
> ble infections, the organization of medical and nursing services
> for the early diagnosis and prevention of disease, the education of
> the individual in personal health, and the *development of the social
> machinery* to assure a standard of living adequate for the mainte-
> nance and improvement of health.[13]

The italicized phrases, *through organized community efforts* and *development of the social machinery,* clearly indicate that participation and civic
engagement were critical components of public health eight decades ago.
Because it is long-standing concept, inseparably linked to the principle of
democracy, rhetoric about the benefits of participation is universal. Yet, in too
many instances, rhetoric about participation is not matched by action. Genuine, collaborative participation is hard, time-consuming work; it has "costs."
It requires us to listen to, and learn about, the ways of others; think of needs
beyond our immediate boundaries; wait longer than we had planned; and
share our power or give up some control.

However, those same costs turn into benefits when we see them as in-
vestments contributing to the development of actions that improve the health
and welfare of the larger community. In this chapter, we have highlighted
some of the core concepts, strategies, and specific tactics that will help practitioners in their ongoing efforts to stimulate public participation, nurture
political support, and heighten the public's awareness of the value of public
health.

ENDNOTES

1. Dall T. *Political Theory and Praxis.* Minneapolis: University of Minnesota
   Press; 1977.
2. World Health Organization. *Alma-Ata 1978: Primary Health Care.* Geneva:
   World Health Organization, "Health for All" Series No. 1.
3. For an in-depth and well-referenced discussion on the principle of participation,
   see Green L. Theory of participation: a qualitative analysis of its expression in
   national and international health policies. In: Ward WB, ed. *Advances in Health
   Education and Promotion.* Greenwich, CT: JAI Press Inc.; 1986: 1(part A):
   211–236.
4. Braithwaite R, Murphy F, Lythcott N, Blumenthal D. Community organization
   and development for health promotion within an urban black community: a
   conceptual model. *Health Educ.* 1989;20(5):56–60.
5. Kretzman J, McKnight J. *Building Communities from the Inside Out.* Chicago:
   ACTA Publications; 1993.
6. Berry W. *What Are People For?* New York: North Point Press; 1990:118–119.

7. Rose G. *The Strategy of Preventive Medicine.* New York: Oxford University Press; 1992:123–124.

8. *Marketing Core Public Health Functions: Summary of Focus Group Findings and Implications for Message Concepts.* Macro International, Inc., and Westat Inc., August 1994. Contract study with the Centers for Disease Control and Prevention #200-93-0653. Practitioners will find this straightforward description a useful resource.

9. Tolsma DD, Koplan JP. Health behaviors and health promotion. In: Last JM, Wallace RB, eds. *Public Health and Preventive Medicine,* 13th ed. East Norwalk, CT: Appleton and Lange; 1992:701–714.

10. Paradoxically, the complexity of multiple audiences is also one of your strongest assets, as it gives you a broader and more diverse base of support that decreases the perception of self-interest. Multiple audiences constitute an advantage to be treasured.

11. As a first point of departure in preparing the plan and content for the seminars, we recommend two rich sources of information: Wallack L, Dorfman L, Jernigan D, Themba M. *Media Advocacy and Public Health.* Newbury Park, CA: Sage Publications; 1993; and Chapman S, Lupton D. *The Fight for Public Health: Principles and Practice of Media Advocacy.* London: BMJ Publishing; 1994.

12. By *decision makers,* we generally mean people who are elected or appointed to government positions such as neighborhood or city councils, boards of county commissioners, and legislatures.

13. Winslow CEA. *The Evolution and Significance of the Modern Public Health Campaign.* New Haven, CT: Yale University Press; 1923. (Reprinted in 1984 by the *Journal of Public Health Policy.*)

CHAPTER 4

What's the Plan?
Is It Working?

WHAT CAUSES THE CAUSES?

Forty tables, six places at each one—and not an empty seat in the house. The tables were covered with starched white cloths, each one topped with two candles and a bouquet of freshly cut flowers. A portable podium centered on a small platform stood at one end of the room, and behind it hung a gold banner with blue letters that read: "Our Kids Count."

The sounds of dinner-table conversation were complemented by the almost unnoticeable background strains of highbrow elevator music. But the entire ambience, including the servers decked out in black and white, could not camouflage the fact that this was the Whitehall Junior High multipurpose room!

The general manager of the new Marriott Hotel had offered the use of one of the hotel's ballrooms at no charge, but the planning committee insisted that the site of the banquet honoring the Our Kids Count Coalition volunteers should be held at the site where it had all started five years ago.

*   *   *

In March 1997, a small group of parents decided to tackle the problem of underage drinking and drug use. They called themselves Villagers Who Care, after the African proverb, "It takes an entire village to raise a child." They joined forces with the Whitehall YMCA, the YWCA, the PTA, and the local cooperative extension office. This new alliance took on the name the Our Kids Count Coalition. Its goal was to plan and sponsor a community workshop on the problem of substance abuse among kids. The workshop was held in the junior high school's multipurpose room and drew 115 participants. The half-day meeting was coordinated by Rachel Warren, the leader of Villagers Who Care. During the first portion of the meeting, specialists from the state departments of education and health presented data comparing national patterns of alcohol, tobacco, and drug use over the past five years with trends seen in the Whitehall area over the same five-year period.

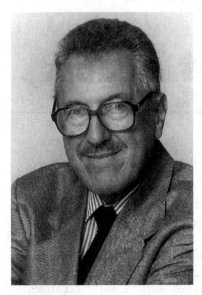

Dr. Dick Loman

Dick Loman, a professor of health education and behavioral science at State University, was featured in the second segment of the workshop. Dr. Loman described the educational, behavioral, and social factors that are usually associated with higher rates of substance abuse. Rachel and other attendees were particularly impressed by the clarity and logic of his presentation. During the four years that followed that first meeting, Dick Loman had played a key role in the development and implementation of the intervention programs supported by the Our Kids Count Coalition.

*   *   *

With few people noticing, Mayor Carl Crawford walked over to the podium. The room quieted as he tapped a spoon against his water glass. He then tapped the microphone with his finger and asked, "Is this working?"

"Yes," the audience responded.

"Evenings like this one make my job worth doing."

A friendly heckler shouted, "Please, no speeches tonight, Mr. Mayor!"

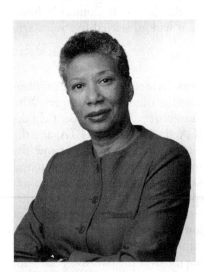

Rachel Warren

Carl laughed. "Not a chance. I want to thank you all for taking the time and effort to join in this celebration. It is inspiring to see this kind of community commitment. At this time, I want to turn the podium over to the champion and president of the Our Kids Count Coalition, Rachel Warren."

The applause was instant, heartfelt, and long. Rachel was simultaneously proud and embarrassed. As she approached the podium, she raised a small booklet and said, "I want to read a passage from this report. It is the 2001 annual report of the task force on substance abuse from our neighboring state, Ohio."

It is probably true that drug dealing and alcohol abuse in suburbia are less likely to occur in plain sight or to cause the neighborhood blight seen in some inner cities. But it is, nevertheless, there. It is hidden, and because it is hidden, it is more insidious. Families with resources and power can harbor secrets about substance abuse that contribute to shame and denial that leads to resistance to action by schools, religious leaders, and sometimes law enforcement.

Rachel added, "We could have written the same thing about Whitehall five years ago, but thanks to your good work"—she gestured by extending her arms toward the audience—"those words are less true today." Rachel paused to pick up another document. "Each of you should have a copy of the latest."

As the banquet guests retrieved their reports, Rachel continued, "The report tells us that, compared to five years ago, our young people are smoking less and consuming less alcohol and other substances; alcohol-related auto crashes are down; and we are seeing better attendance in schools and fewer dropouts. Although we would like to have seen even larger differences, and we still have a long road ahead, the truth is that we are making a difference!"

The burst of applause was spontaneous. When it subsided, Rachel said, "We could not have accomplished what we have without the unselfish commitment of those of you whom we honor tonight: our wonderful corps of volunteers. Now, I would like Mayor Crawford to return to the podium and, with the able assistance of Bobbie Washington, student body president of Whitehall Senior High (who, I might add, is one of our youth volunteers), make the formal presentation of awards. Mr. Mayor?"

As the awards were being presented, Rachel thought of Dick Loman and wished that he could have been there. He had moved away from the area one year before to take a new position in the Division of Adolescent and School Health at the Centers for Disease Control and Prevention in Atlanta. It had been Dick who, four years earlier, had provided the insight and leadership for bringing a much-needed focus to the coalition's planning process.

The Our Kids Count Coalition had been formed about three months after the initial workshop in March 1997. The new coalition was fueled by two sources of energy: (1) the recognition that substance abuse was a serious threat to the quality of life of Whitehall, and (2) the astute and passionate leadership of Rachel Warren, whose most obvious attribute was, paradoxically, that "just saying no" to her was not an option!

During the latter part of its first year, the coalition began preparations to submit a grant application for funding support from the Center for Substance Abuse Prevention (CSAP) in the U.S. Department of Health and Human Services. The Whitehall school board had agreed to join the coalition as the fiscal agent in the grant application.

As they undertook the background work necessary to prepare the application, some coalition members wondered if they hadn't underestimated just how complex and multidimensional the problem of substance abuse was. It was difficult for some to see just how they were going to get their arms around such a complicated issue. But Rachel had an idea!

She remembered the presentation Dick Loman had given at that initial workshop in March 1997. Rachel got in touch with him by phone at the university. She described the goals of the Our Kids Count Coalition and explained that, in close cooperation with the Whitehall school district, the coalition was seeking a CSAP grant. Dick indicated that he was quite familiar with the CSAP grant process. Next, Rachel explained that a small work group had the responsibility for preparing the grant application and, pending a grant award, continuing in that advisory capacity. However, as they got further into the task, it had become clear to Rachel that the group needed technical assistance in bringing its application into sharper focus. Rachel and Dick worked out a plan wherein Dick would meet with the work group for the purpose of grounding them in two critical processes: (1) data-driven, diagnostic planning and (2) accountability or evaluation.

Two weeks later, Rachel and five members of the coalition grant application work group got together with Dick at a conference room at the Whitehall Department of Health for a half-day meeting. As he was being introduced to members of the work group, Dick was pleasantly surprised to find that an old friend, Al Freeman, was among them. Al had been a curriculum coordinator for the state department of education and had recently taken a position as assistant principal at Whitehall Senior High. Audrey Maxfield, Director of the Whitehall Social Services Department; Jane Keller, with the Whitehall YWCA; Juvenile Court Judge Gene Matthews; and Greg Widders, manager of the local Home Depot, were the other members of the workgroup.

Before the group gathered formally, Dick asked Al whether Whitehall was one of the communities covered in the surveys that the state department of education had been conducting since 1990 on students' knowledge, attitudes, and practices related to substance abuse. Al confirmed that Whitehall was indeed part of the sample and indicated that the coalition had plans to make good use of the data.

At Dick's request, Rachel began the meeting by providing a quick briefing on the coalition's vision, goals, membership, and major activities to date. When she had completed her briefing, Rachel turned the floor over to Dr. Loman. Dick thanked Rachel and told the members of the work group that, from his perspective, they had a lot going for them. Then, he turned to a flip chart and unveiled four specific accomplishments that the group had made. (See Figure 4.1.)

Dick noted that all of those accomplishments would be pluses in their application. He then began to explain some of the key things grant review panels typically look for.

"Keep in mind who typically serves on government review panels: they are 'experts,' most of whom are university types. They are on the lookout for

1. Defined the problem: unacceptable levels of substance abuse by youth.

2. Made a clear case showing the many ways in which substance abuse compromises the quality of life of Whitehall: school dropouts and absenteeism, crime, vehicular injuries, and death.

3. Received firm commitments from the local school district and multiple community agencies and organizations to support a comprehensive strategy.

4. Acquired access to data and information that would enable them to track whether changes were occurring.

FIGURE 4.1   Accomplishments of the Our Kids Count Coalition

evidence that the circumstances surrounding the problem being addressed are well documented and clearly defined. They favor sound logic and tend to be leery of proposals that are grandiose or 'pie in the sky.' If you indicate that one of your objectives is to improve (or change in a positive direction) the attitudes and practices of kids age 12 to 16 in Whitehall, they will want to know specifically what attitudes and what practices you are talking about! They will also want to see some justification for selecting those specific attitudes and practices."

Dick paused, and then added, "Rachel told me earlier that the coalition was taking some steps to strengthen the enforcement of laws pertaining to alcohol and tobacco sales to youth. That is also a plus, because when you indicate that you are proposing to implement new policies or strengthen existing ones, you will be able to answer two of the questions the review panel will ask: Policies about what? To accomplish what end?" Members of the work group nodded, acknowledging the points Dick was making.

Then he said, "And finally, if I were a member of the panel, I would ask you this: Keeping in mind your overall goal, if you could accomplish only a portion of the things you propose, which would be the most important?"

Judge Matthews quickly responded, "Enforcing the sales-to-minors laws. You don't use what you don't have."

Al Freeman responded, "There's no question that we do need to enforce existing policies, but we can't stop there. We need a much better educational program for everyone in the community—not just for the kids."

Sounding very much like an attorney, Judge Matthews responded, "He asked which would be the *most important* thing, not the *only* thing."

Dick Loman then called on his teaching experience. "You're right, Judge. I was trying to make the point that you will have to address the matter of setting priorities, because it is highly unlikely that you will have either the time or the resources to do all of the things you want to do." The judge smiled.

Dick continued, "On the other hand, Al has made an equally important point. To achieve your vision, you will need a strategy consisting of the right mix of activities and programs. Policy is sure to be a critical component, but what else will need to be in place if you are to realize your goal?

"I took the liberty of creating an example illustrating a framework or model that many program planners and researchers have found helpful in answering the kind of questions I've just raised." He flipped to a new page. "I want to walk you through this diagram to give you a feel for how the model works. As we go through this process, imagine that we are trying to answer the question: What causes the causes?" (See Figure 4.2.)

"In the box to your far right, numbered 1, we've stated a specific behavior of interest—in this case, youth (12 to 14 years of age) refusing to drink alcohol at a party. Incidentally, the process I am about to describe applies whether you are trying to understand individual behaviors—that is, one student or one patient—or collective behavior—that is, a group or community. Boxes 2, 3, 4, and 5 represent categories of different factors that have the potential of influencing that specific behavior.

"To make this simple, I am going to walk through this example as if our target is a 14-year-old named Rusty. Realistically, we would apply the principles of this process to a broad sampling of youth aged 12 to 14 who reside in Whitehall. The factors in box 2 pertain to the knowledge, attitudes, and beliefs that can influence a given action.

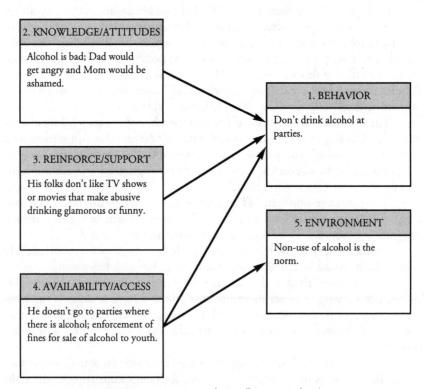

FIGURE 4.2   Factors That Influence Behavior

"The hypothetical information about Rusty indicates that he knows that alcohol can impair his judgment and that it is against the law for him to drink alcohol. He also believes that if his dad found out that he drank, he'd be in big trouble, and if his mom found out, she'd be ashamed.

"Box 3 calls our attention to those factors that reward or reinforce a given action. Let's say that Rusty's parents express their dismay, rather than humor, over films or TV shows that portray episodes of out-of-control drinking as glamorous or funny, and that his best friends behave in ways that suggest they think drinking is stupid.

"Box 4 asks us to consider the matters of availability and accessibility. Suppose that alcohol is rarely, if ever, available at parties that Rusty attends and that older peers and adult vendors with whom he comes in contact don't even think about making alcohol available to him or his friends.

"Box 5 contains factors that represent forces in the social environment.[1] In this instance, a variety of weekend and after-school social programs are available for youth in Rusty's age group, including athletic leagues run by police and religious groups."

With a straight face, Jane Keller said, "Sounds like Rusty lives in *Mister Rogers' Neighborhood!*" Everyone laughed, including Dick, who added rhetorically, "Too good to be true, eh?"

He went to the flip chart, took out a red marking pen, drew a line through the references to Rusty's beliefs about his parents' reactions described in box 2, and wrote in "Drinking is cool." Then he pointed to box 3 and said, "Instead of what we have here, suppose I had put something like this: Rusty's parents, like most parents in the community, are dead set against 'hard' drugs but don't think drinking a 'few beers' is all that bad. After all, they did it when they were young."

He then focused his attention on box 4, speaking as he wrote, "One of his best friends often drinks on weekends, and alcohol and tobacco are easily gotten from convenience stores."

Greg Widders spoke up, "So much for *Mister Rogers' Neighborhood!*"

"Exactly," Dick answered. "Suppose we analyzed the data we have on youth aged 12 to 14 in Whitehall, and the profile we came up with was similar to this last adjustment we made on the example with Rusty. How would this knowledge influence the way you allocate your resources? Would you direct them to programs teaching kids about the dangers of alcohol abuse? Or to programs teaching skills that kids need to resist pressure from friends? Or to programs aimed at creating heightened awareness among parents—especially of how their behavior affects kids? Or to establishing and enforcing sales-to-minors laws?"

Judge Matthews mused out loud, "This way of assessing the situation makes it clear that doing just one thing is not likely to get the job, yet we have to grapple with time and resource limits. This is a tough problem—we have some tough choices to make!"

Dick pointed out that the kind of assessment he was describing was part of the Precede–Proceed planning process[2] that is widely used to help planners with those "tough choices" by bringing to light those factors that, if effectively addressed, would most likely lead to the health improvement goal being sought. He then observed that Henry David Thoreau once said, "'there are thousands hacking at the branches of evil to one who is striking at the root.' The logic of an assessment process like this is to help you get as close to those roots as possible."

Dick then set the stage for the segment on evaluation by asking the work group members to imagine for a moment that their grant application was successful. "Now let's look two or three years down the road. How likely is it that you will have, to your satisfaction, effectively addressed the youth substance abuse problem in Whitehall?"

Jane Keller was the first to respond. "I think it will be possible to show some progress but I also think it is unrealistic to expect to see dramatic changes."

"I agree with Jane," said Greg Widders. "I also think it would be important to clarify what we mean when we say this or that will be done 'to our satisfaction.' For example, in the business world small changes are important. We frequently use the concept of market shares—which refers to the portion of given products sold in a given year achieved by a given brand—say, power saws. If we increase our current market share of power saws sales by 4–5 percent, that would be big!"

"So while we should expect to be able to make progress, we shouldn't expect that difference to be a spectacular one in just two years. We also need to be clear on what constitutes success and what measures we're going to use to determine the degree of success." Dick asked, "Is that a fair summary?"

"I'd like to add one more point," said Audrey Maxfield. "Since I became director of social services, my board has been tenacious about the notion of accountability. Few board meetings go by where board members do not ask for examples of progress we are making or the problems we've encountered. They also want to know how we addressed those problems and how we are managing our budget."

Dick asked Audrey if being held accountable had been a hassle. According to Audrey, at first the structure and process was intimidating. Now, however, she considered it a blessing because it put staff expectations in sync with those of the board and kept all of the stakeholders focused.

Dick observed that the group's comments were all examples of practical, real-world examples of the importance of evaluation. He assured the group that the panelists who would be reviewing the grant application would surely want a clear signal from the people in Whitehall on what they expected to achieve and when they expected to achieve it. The team would also want to know the kind of evidence that Whitehall planned to use to document its level of achievement. Dick pointed out that the critical elements of evaluation were, in effect, built into the planning process, in the form of careful assessment and the delineation of measurable objectives.

The ensuing discussion was both lively and productive. Dick gave several examples of how the work group could apply this diagnostic planning approach, using existing data from Whitehall, to propose multiple, and measurable, strategies in the grant application. The group members, in turn, felt as if Dick Loman's counsel had helped them put the complexity of their challenge into a more realistic perspective.

The next morning, Dick called Rachel and accepted her invitation to join the work group. In the ensuing weeks, he recruited two graduate students, who subsequently helped design and administer a questionnaire to collect information that would fill in a few information gaps. The work group completed the grant application on time.

Five months after Dick Loman's workshop with the work group, the Whitehall school district and the Our Kids Count Coalition were officially notified that they had received a $1.3 million grant from CSAP.

* * *

After the last volunteer had been recognized, Mayor Crawford asked those gathered for one last round of appreciation. Rachel thought to herself, "Dick Loman would have liked this."

Case Analysis

In the "What Causes the Causes?" case story, we can see that the Our Kids Count Coalition evolved into a force to be reckoned with in Whitehall. Under Rachel's strong leadership, the coalition helped to heighten social consciousness about alcohol and drug abuse and, in doing so, inspired communitywide hope that better things were ahead for the young people of Whitehall. Their pursuit of the CSAP grant forced coalition members to express their hopes in more tangible terms. That process brought into sharper relief both the magnitude and complexity of the problem they were taking on—initially, some coalition members had feared that they would not be able to get a handle on a problem as complex as substance abuse.

When Dr. Loman provided the example of the diagnostic planning model, he helped members of the work group see a way to get not one but several "handles" on the problem. He also helped them see the utility of probing for the factors that explain why substance abuse was a problem in Whitehall because it would give them the essential information they needed to make informed decisions about specific activities or programs.

In addition, these probes encouraged coalition members to examine and describe the logic behind their choices—information that would be helpful not only in guiding their selection of potential intervention strategies, but also in developing an evaluation plan. The remainder of this chapter provides the details one should attend to when applying this approach to program planning and evaluation.

ASSUMPTIONS

Before practitioners get to the point where they will be applying the process that follows, we must make several assumptions:

Assumption 1: A "shared vision" has already been established for the overall program.

Assumption 2: A specific health problem has been identified and a measurable health objective has been stated.

Assumption 3: One of the program's priority tasks is to identify social/environmental conditions and behaviors that are (1) known to contribute to the health problem in question and (2) amenable to change.

Assumption 4: The program has limited time and resources.

THE TARGETS FOR CHANGE

Over the years, health promotion practitioners in school, community, clinical, and workplace settings, like Dick Loman in the case story, have found the Precede–Proceed model to be a valuable tool for solving a variety of complex problems. In the portion of the Precede–Proceed model emphasized here, we start with the task given in Assumption 3: to identify social/environmental conditions and behaviors that are (1) known to contribute to the health problem in question and (2) amenable to change. Suppose that your planning group has drafted the following overall program objective:

> By the year 2000, as a result of a coordinated prevention program, reduce fatal injuries among those aged 15 to 24 caused by motor vehicle crashes in [your community] to no more than 17 per 100,000 population. (The current local rate is 33 per 100,000.)

Once the program objective has been established, here are the steps you would follow to get a clearer picture of the specific actions you might take to achieve that objective.

Step 1: List Risk Factors

Use your knowledge of the relevant literature and your past experience to generate a list of the potential behavioral and environmental factors known to be risk factors for motor vehicle injuries. Your list might include the following items:

Use of seat belts	Air bags in car
Driver's age	Road conditions

Weather conditions

Driving ability

Heavy traffic

Street lighting

Illegal sale of alcohol to minors

Driving speed

Driver's gender

Speed limits

Driving under the influence
  of alcohol

Child safety seat usage

Location of crash

Time/day of week when crashes occur

Placement of warning signs

Laws prohibiting alcohol sales to
  minors not enforced

Step 2: Differentiate Between Behavioral and Environmental Factors

Examine the list and determine which factors are behavioral and which are environmental. In this case, simply place a *B* for behavioral or an *E* for environmental next to each factor.

_____ Use of seat belts

_____ Driver's age

_____ Air bags in car

_____ Road conditions

_____ Weather conditions

_____ Driving ability

_____ Heavy traffic

_____ Street lighting

_____ Illegal sale of alcohol
         to minors

_____ Driving speed

_____ Driver's gender

_____ Speed limits

_____ Driving under the influence
         of alcohol

_____ Child safety seat usage

_____ Location of crash

_____ Time/day of week when
         crashes occur

_____ Placement of warning signs

_____ Laws prohibiting alcohol
         sales to minors not enforced

This may seem a tedious process. But the investment in time now can save you time later and help you avoid the frustrating and sometimes embarrassing experience of having to do it all over again!

Step 3: Shorten the List

Remember, the purpose of this process is to help you focus on those key factors that will help you achieve your program objective. The key question is this: What criteria should you use to winnow the list down? By definition, practitioners are practical. They want to do things that count, things that are relevant. In this process, therefore, there is an ever-present question: Which of these factors apply in this specific situation?

In addition to drawing on the experience they have gained by working with the population in question, practitioners will find rich sources of community-specific information in records kept by local police, emergency medical services, and the results of local surveys and focus-group interviews. Suppose that such local information confirms that the following six factors are relevant to the current example:

- Use of seat belts
- Driving speed
- Driving under the influence of alcohol
- Age of driver
- Driving ability
- Location of crash

To create an even more manageable list, the next step is to reexamine the factors and determine the extent to which each is important and changeable.

Step 4: Determine Factor Importance

To determine the *importance* of a given factor, you need to answer two questions:

1. How prevalent is the behavior, or how frequently is the environmental factor involved?
2. Does good evidence exist showing that the factor clearly contributes to the health problem?

Based on the information we have available to answer these questions, Figure 4.3 shows how we would rate each factor along a continuum from "More Important" to "Less Important."

Note: If your planning circumstances enable you to engage multiple experts or participants in the rating process, we would recommend creating a 10-point scale along the continuum. Ask each of the raters to identify a specific number, and then add the numbers and average the ratings. Those items scoring above the midpoint of the scale can be treated as more important; those scoring below the midpoint should be considered less important.

Step 5: Determine Changeability

Health promotion practitioners are charged with developing programs that will "make a difference." In most instances, that difference will be reflected in

More Important   **Use of Seat Belts**   Less Important

```
  └──x──────────────────────────────────────────────────────────────┘
```

Comment: Seat belts are used by only 27 percent of drivers involved in crashes.

More Important   **Driving Speed**   Less Important

```
  └────────────────────────────────────────────x─────────────────────┘
```

Comment: In crashes not involving alcohol, excess speed is a factor in only 3 percent of the cases.

More Important   **Drinking and Driving**   Less Important

```
  └x─────────────────────────────────────────────────────────────────┘
```

Comment: Forty-four percent of all motor vehicle fatalities are alcohol related; a local survey shows that 50 percent of high-school youth report that they have either driven while drinking or been with a driver who has been drinking.

More Important   **Age of Driver**   Less Important

```
  └──x────────────────────────────────────────────────────────────────┘
```

Comment: Forty-eight percent of motor vehicle crashes involve drivers under age 19.

More Important   **Sales to Minors**   Less Important

```
  └───x────────────────────────────────────────────────────────────────┘
```

Comment: A recent school-based survey of self-reported behaviors indicated that when minors try to purchase cigarettes from selected quick-stop stores or older friends, they are successful three out of four times.

More Important   **Enforcement of Laws re: Sales to Minors**   Less Important

```
  └───x────────────────────────────────────────────────────────────────┘
```

Comment: Police records reveal that there have been no charges brought against local merchants for sale of alcoholic beverages to minors in the last three years.

FIGURE 4.3   Rating Environmental Factors by Importance

a measurable change in a specific behavior or environmental condition. Because some behaviors and environmental factors are more or less changeable, knowledge of changeability will help the practitioner not only determine the feasibility of "making a difference," but also estimate the time it will take to detect a difference.

As an example, suppose we have two groups of smokers. One group consists of teenagers in Des Moines, Iowa, all of whom began smoking within the past year. The other group includes men who live in Budapest, Hungary, all of whom are older than 40 and have been smoking their entire adult lives. While the possibility of change exists for both groups, the effort and time needed to change the latter group would be far greater than that for the former!

Change is more likely to occur when a behavior is in the early developmental stages or has been adopted only recently, and when there is some expression of willingness to change on the part of the individual or group.[3] As we all know from our own life experiences, change is more difficult when the action has been long established, when it is deeply rooted in cultural practices and beliefs, when prior efforts to change have been ineffective, and when there is evidence that the individual or group in question has no interest in making a change.

Our experience is that determining the potential for change among environmental factors is less amenable to prescription, and that the practitioner needs to rely on good judgment. Here are a few simple rules of thumb we have found helpful. Changeability is likely to be high if:

- There are precedents elsewhere for similar changes.

  Example: As a part of a communitywide cardiovascular disease prevention program in Wichita, Kansas, the program director wants to increase the number of restaurants that offer low-fat menu options and provide no-smoking seating areas. Similar efforts have been successful in Kansas City.

- The economic costs are not prohibitive.

  Example: Inordinately high rates of injury and death among seniors in Brooklyn, New York, have been attributed to the following cause: senior pedestrians have been hit by motor vehicles while trying to cross a wide street (Queens Boulevard), especially during the morning and afternoon rush hours. The majority of senior pedestrians are unable to cross Queens Boulevard in the time allotted for the green light. The light-change timing pattern has been lengthened, and speed bumps have been installed in the area.

- The proposed change is supported by public demand.

  Example: Most observers agree that a significant part of the success of the well-documented North Karelia Project can be attributed to its ability to educate the public and thereby create a public demand for the food industry to increase its production of skim milk, low-fat dairy products, and fruits and vegetables.

Based on the information we have, Figure 4.4 shows how we would position each of the previously mentioned factors along a continuum from "More Changeable" to "Less Changeable."

Step 6: Create a Matrix

Information from your importance and changeability analyses (Figures 4.3 and 4.4) will enable you to create a single "picture" in the form of a simple 2-by-2 matrix like the one shown in Figure 4.5. Using the same ratings applied on each continuum, the matrix reveals how the various factors "cluster" in terms of importance and changeability.

The factors that end up in quadrant 1 are those that are both important and changeable. As such, they are likely to be prime targets for your health promotion program. In this example, the age of the driver is deemed important but less changeable and, therefore, is placed in quadrant 2. The rating of high importance was made based on the fact that nearly half of all crashes involved drivers under the age of 19.

Although one cannot literally change age, figuratively it is changeable in the sense that the minimum age for obtaining a driver's license might be changed from the current 16 years of age to 18. Eliminating the rule permitting earlier licensing if a teenager takes a driver education course is one way of changing the average age of drivers.

In most instances, factors deemed highly important but less changeable are good targets for an innovative intervention if accompanied by careful evaluation. Evidence from such evaluations that a new approach can change a given factor could then be used to argue for greater changeability and wider application of that approach.

For example, suppose you are planning a program designed to reduce sexual promiscuity and unprotected sex among a culturally diverse population of teens. You read an article by Dan Romer and his colleagues,[6] which describes a strategy wherein a group of parents in an African American neighborhood shared the responsibility for monitoring the actions of children and youth within their "friendship network." The effect of this approach was a marked reduction in sexual activity. You acknowledge the importance of parental supervision, and this approach makes good intuitive sense to you. Nevertheless, you can't be certain how feasible it would be to implement such a strategy in the population you are serving. In that case, you would likely list "Parental Monitoring" in quadrant 2 and make certain that the appropriate steps are taken to assess the extent to which this activity (1) was properly implemented and (2) had an effect on your program objective.

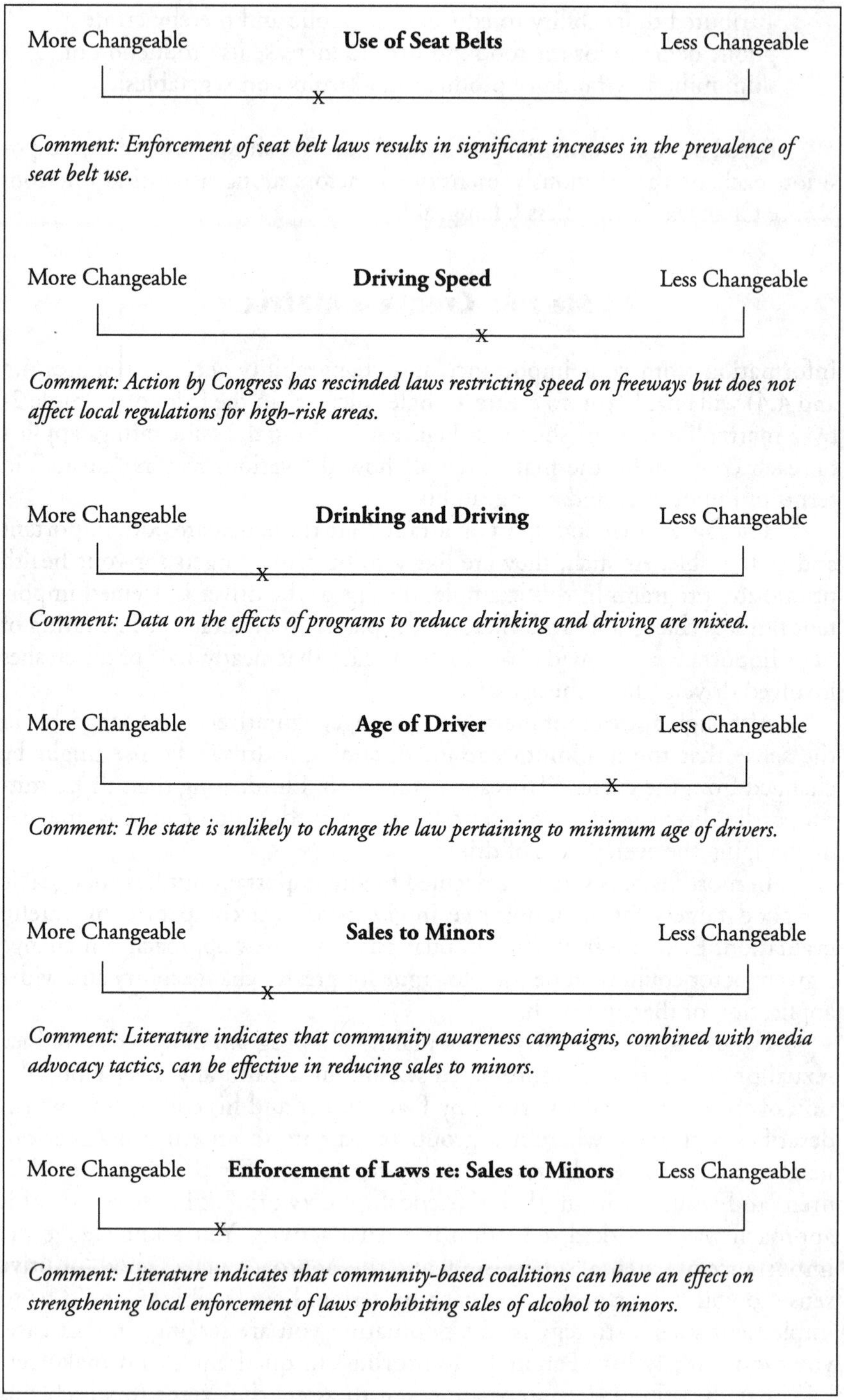

More Changeable   **Use of Seat Belts**   Less Changeable

Comment: Enforcement of seat belt laws results in significant increases in the prevalence of seat belt use.

More Changeable   **Driving Speed**   Less Changeable

Comment: Action by Congress has rescinded laws restricting speed on freeways but does not affect local regulations for high-risk areas.

More Changeable   **Drinking and Driving**   Less Changeable

Comment: Data on the effects of programs to reduce drinking and driving are mixed.

More Changeable   **Age of Driver**   Less Changeable

Comment: The state is unlikely to change the law pertaining to minimum age of drivers.

More Changeable   **Sales to Minors**   Less Changeable

Comment: Literature indicates that community awareness campaigns, combined with media advocacy tactics, can be effective in reducing sales to minors.

More Changeable   **Enforcement of Laws re: Sales to Minors**   Less Changeable

Comment: Literature indicates that community-based coalitions can have an effect on strengthening local enforcement of laws prohibiting sales of alcohol to minors.

FIGURE 4.4   Rating Environmental Factors by Changeability

	More Important	Less Important
More Changeable	• Drinking and Driving • Sales to Minors • Enforcement of Laws • Use of Seat Belts Quadrant 1	• Driving Speed Quadrant 3
Less Changeable	• Age of Driver Quadrant 2	 Quadrant 4

FIGURE 4.5   Importance and Changeability Matrix

Step 7: Set Objectives

The potential effectiveness of a health promotion program can be jeopardized when the objectives are stated in vague language and thus are difficult to measure. Given the assumption that practitioners have limited time and resources, vagueness is not a prudent option. When behavior change is deemed important and possible, care must be taken to state objectives with care and precision. Such objectives should answer these questions:

Who? (the people expected to change)

What? (the action or change to be achieved)

How much? (the extent of the condition to be achieved)

When? (the time in which the change is expected to occur)

Here are sample objectives for two of the factors that appear in quadrant 1 of Figure 4.5:

- **Drinking and Driving** (behavioral factor). By September 2000, we will reduce by 50 percent the number of youth aged 16 to 18 who report that they drink and drive.

- **Sales to Minors** (environmental factor). By June 1998, local government authorities will implement and actively support a policy calling for full enforcement of laws prohibiting sales of alcohol to minors.

IDENTIFYING THE CAUSES

Once the priority behavioral and environmental objectives have been determined, planners need to answer this question: What factors seem to be contributing to the behavioral and environmental conditions that they seek to influence? Once those candidates have been identified, many of the steps used to determine importance and changeability will be repeated.

We make the assumption that all behavioral and environmental targets are shaped by a variety of factors and conditions, some of which are likely to have a greater influence on outcomes than others. This variety reflects the complexity that is inherent when dealing with any human/social problem. Accountable health promotion practitioners cannot deny that complexity; they can only work within it. A portion of the Precede–Proceed model includes a graphic framework to help practitioners manage that complexity. Figure 4.6 provides an illustration of that framework.

Predisposing factors help practitioners to cluster and examine how cognitive capacities (what we know) and affective characteristics (how we feel

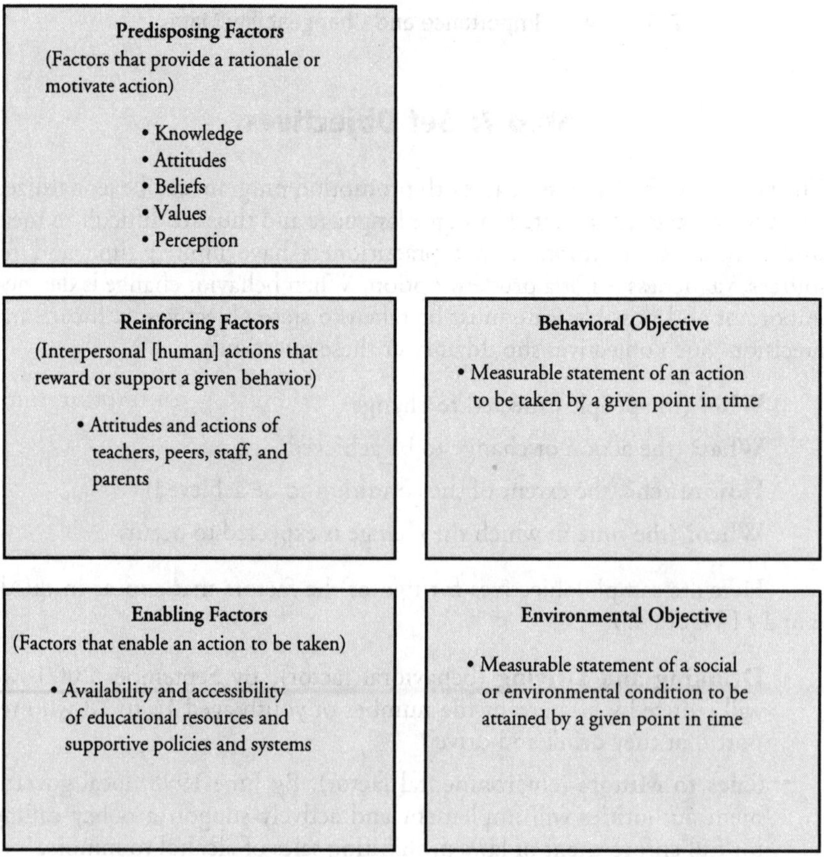

Predisposing Factors
(Factors that provide a rationale or motivate action)

- Knowledge
- Attitudes
- Beliefs
- Values
- Perception

Reinforcing Factors
(Interpersonal [human] actions that reward or support a given behavior)

- Attitudes and actions of teachers, peers, staff, and parents

Behavioral Objective

- Measurable statement of an action to be taken by a given point in time

Enabling Factors
(Factors that enable an action to be taken)

- Availability and accessibility of educational resources and supportive policies and systems

Environmental Objective

- Measurable statement of a social or environmental condition to be attained by a given point in time

FIGURE 4.6 Predisposing, Reinforcing, and Enabling Factors

and what we believe in) might influence a specific pattern of behavior. For example, (1) the absence of knowledge, (2) the belief that one has no control over what happens to him or her, and (3) feelings of low self-confidence regarding changing the behavior in question are modifiable characteristics that can put an individual or group at unnecessary risk.

We have often heard the comment that when it comes right down to it, knowledge plays a very small role in influencing behavior. An example of this attitude might be the following: "Teen smokers will not give up their habit just because you tell them they will be 20 times more likely to die from lung cancer than those who don't smoke by the time they reach age 55." While this example is a good one, it does not merit the generalization that knowledge is comparatively unimportant.

Suppose you have been assigned to work in a region of Nigeria where malaria is the leading cause of death and disability. It has been determined that pockets of standing water, which could be readily cleaned up, are the primary breeding grounds for mosquitoes. To what extent would a culturally sensitive understanding of this knowledge be of importance to the villagers and their leaders?

The point we wish to make is this: The value of an analytic process like the one we are using here is that it asks practitioners to assess the reality and circumstances under which they are working. Depending upon that reality, knowledge may or may not be a critical factor; such a decision can be made only after thoughtful review.

Some practitioners refer to **reinforcing factors** in terms of the notion of feedback. That fits! Reinforcement is feedback with effect; feedback rewards the action taken. The attitudes and climate of support one gets (or doesn't get) can have a very strong influence on behavior. Thus, it should be a priority to determine the role that parents, family members, co-workers, peers, best friends, health care providers, supervisors, and other people play in supporting or discouraging a given behavior. Because exposure to the media also falls into this category, similar consideration should be given to print, film, and electronic media, including the Internet.

Those conditions of the environment that facilitate actions by individuals, groups, or organizations are called **enabling factors**. The extent to which services, facilities, programs, or program elements are available, accessible, and/or affordable are good examples of this factor. Negative examples include the following:

- Encouraging low-income women over age 50 to seek mammograms while failing to take into account that mammograms are (1) available only during hours that the women are working and (2) unaffordable for them

- Promoting a tobacco-use prevention and control program for youth without addressing the reality that tobacco vending machines are ubiquitous

Also included under this category are the specific skills one needs to perform a given behavior. For example, a health promotion program designed to enhance the strength and flexibility of senior citizens must take into account the skills and capacity of the participants to execute the prescribed exercises and activities. Failure to acknowledge the importance of those skills could lead to unrealistic expectations, which in turn could negatively affect self-esteem and discourage participation.

GENERATING PREDISPOSING, REINFORCING, AND ENABLING FACTORS

To get a sense of how to apply this level of analysis, let's return to one of the objectives stated earlier:

- By September 2000, we will reduce by 50 percent the number of youth aged 16 to 18 who report that they drink and drive.

Step 1. Generate a list of factors that may affect or explain why young people in your community choose to drink and drive.

- Teens do not perceive themselves to be at risk: "It won't happen to me."
- Police know the likely days/times of crashes, but don't patrol.
- The media glamorize beer.
- The mayor thinks teen drinking and driving is an important issue.
- Eighty-five percent of teens report that they know the dangers of drinking and driving.
- Many parents believe that taking drugs, not drinking alcohol, is the problem.
- Alcohol at teen parties is a tradition.
- Laws prohibiting sales to minors are not enforced.

Step 2. Classify these items as predisposing, reinforcing, or enabling factors. Figure 4.7 presents an illustration of how the factors generated in Step 1 fall into the three categories.

The remainder of the process follows exactly the same steps you followed in the previous exercise.

Step 3. Using the same criteria you applied earlier, determine the importance of each factor.

Step 4. Repeat the same process to determine the changeability of each factor.

Step 5. Create a matrix to help you visualize the factors that have the highest importance and changeability ratings.

Step 6. For each factor on which you chose to focus, state a measurable objective that incorporates the essential elements of this question: *Who will do how much of what by when?*

Predisposing Factors
• Teens do not perceive themselves to be at risk: "It won't happen to me." • Merchants do not think they will be prosecuted for selling alcohol to minors.

Reinforcing Factors	Behavioral Objective
• Many parents believe that drugs, not alcohol, are the problem. • Laws prohibiting sales to minors are not enforced. • The media glamorize beer. • The mayor thinks teen drinking and driving is an important issue.	• By September 2000, we will reduce by 50 percent the number of youth aged 16 to 18 who report that they drink and drive.

Enabling Factors	Environmental Objective
• Alcohol at teen parties is a tradition. • It is easy to buy alcohol.	• Reduce sales of alcohol to minors by 50 percent by 1999.

FIGURE 4.7   Factors That Influence Teen Drinking and Driving

G'DAY: AUSTRALIA'S DIAGNOSTIC APPROACH

This diagnostic process has been used in literally hundreds of applications around the world. In 1996, we had the opportunity to visit a project under way in Western Australia, where researchers at Curtin University and local school officials in Perth were working on an intervention to reduce child pedestrian injuries, the leading cause of death and severe injury in children in Western Australia. In the office where the central planning for the project was carried out, a modified version of this diagnostic approach was posted on the wall as a large working flow chart; the Australian group used this flow chart to keep members of the team focused on their specific tasks within the context of the overall program strategy. With permission from the Australian researchers and practitioners directing that project, we have recreated that chart as Tables 4.1 and 4.2. As you scan the tables, notice how they have clearly delineated the behavioral factors (Table 4.1) and environmental

TABLE 4.1 Preventing Pedestrian Injuries Among Five- to Nine-Year-Olds

Behavioral Factors	Contributing Factors	Intervention Strategy Selection
RF *Children crossing roads* **O** Reduce percentage of children crossing at busy roads **O** Increase percentage of children crossing at safer sites	*Belief of children—low perception of risk re: crossing busy roads* **SO** Develop beliefs of children *Lack of environmental supports* **SO** ID safer sites *Knowledge of children re: road-crossing behaviors (RCB)* **SO** Enhance knowledge of children	**StO** School education: 1. develop beliefs of children re: risk of crossing busy roads 2. ID alternative "safer" routes, map routes, etc. 3. ID "safer" crossing sites **StO** Parent education on child pedestrian safety **StO** Environmental: improve signs, paint curbs, increase number of crossing attendants
RF *Inappropriate crossing behavior by 5- to 9-year-olds* **O** Improve children's road-crossing behaviors **O** Improve children's "search" behaviors	*Beliefs of children—perception of invulnerability, etc.* **SO** Develop beliefs of children *Road-crossing skills of children* **SO** Enhance road-crossing skills of children *Inadequate family modeling of RCB* **SO** Improve family modeling	**StO** Create action/experience/modeling school pedestrian safety education program **StO** Provide teacher training and follow-up support to ensure implementation of the school pedestrian safety education program **StO** Create a parent pedestrian safety education program
RF *Children not getting help to cross roads* **O** Increase percentage of children getting help to cross roads	*Inadequate school-based road safety education* **SO** Implement quality road safety education *Parents' perceptions of children's abilities to cross roads safely* **SO** Change parents' perceptions	**StO** Create action/experience/modeling school pedestrian safety education program

Lack of supervision of children by parents

SO Improve appropriate supervision by parents

Social skills (decision making, assertive communication) demonstrated by children when asking people to help them cross roads

SO Enhance social skills of children

Parent perceptions of child's abilities to cross roads safely

SO Change parents' perceptions

StO Create a parent pedestrian safety education program

RF *Parents not supervising children at crossings*

O Increase percentage of parents supervising children at road crossings

RF *Parents not teaching appropriate road-crossing procedures*

O Increase percentage of parents teaching children appropriate road-crossing procedures

RF *Parents not modeling appropriate road-crossing behaviors*

O Increase percentage of parents modeling appropriate road-crossing behaviors

Legend:
RF = risk factor
O = objective
SO = subobjective
StO = strategic objective

TABLE 4.2 Environmental Factors: Volume and Speed of Traffic, Road Design, Roadside Obstacles

	Environmental Factors	Contributing Factors	Intervention Strategy
RF	*High volume of traffic on residential streets*	*Posted residential speed limits too high*	**StO** *Inform council and state government
O	Reduce residential traffic volume (% reduction in traffic volume, construction of speed control measures)	**SO** Reduce posted residential speed limit	**StO** Inform council to redesign and replan roads
		Road design in residential areas encourages speeding and high traffic volume	**StO** Inform police to enforce residential speed limits
RF	*Speed of vehicles too fast on residential streets*	**SO** Change road design	**StO** Develop community education campaign/ programs
O	Reduce speed of vehicles (% reduction in average speed)	**SO** Council to redesign and replan	
		Drivers exceeding posted speed limit — lack of enforcement	
		SO Police to enforce residential speed limits	
		Beliefs of drivers — low perception of being caught by police or causing injury	
		SO Change beliefs of drivers	
		Knowledge of drivers re: children's road-crossing capabilities, etc.	
		SO Change knowledge of drivers	
		Lack of community road safety education	
		SO Develop community road safety program	

102

RF *Road design exposes children to busy roads*
O Redesign road hierarchy to reduce traffic volume
(% reduction in traffic volume—changes in road hierarchy)

RF *Road hierarchy design encourages speeding in residential areas*
O Redesign road hierarchy to reduce traffic speed on local streets
(% reduction in traffic speed—changes in road hierarchy)

Road hierarchy designs need coordination
SO State government to modify road hierarchy plan
SO Council to redesign and replan roads

Road design in residential areas encourages speeding and traffic volume
SO Change road design

StO Inform state government re: road hierarchy plan
StO Inform council to redesign and replan

RF *Roadside obstacles obscuring children*
O Reduce obscuring obstacles
O Relocate/redesign structures (posts/booths)
O Restrict parking/alternative parking

Knowledge or perception of council staff and community about roadside obstacles
SO Change knowledge/perception of council staff and community

StO Develop community education campaign/programs
StO Inform staff/authorities, etc.

Legend:
RF = risk factor
O = objective
SO = subobjective
StO = strategic objective
*Inform through advocacy and information campaigns

factors (Table 4.2). Note, too, that the interventions described cover a wide range of coordinated educational, environmental, regulatory, and enforcement strategies. All of the information displayed in the two tables represents practical examples of how indicators are used to inform the evaluation process.

EVALUATION: STAYING ON COURSE

Prior to setting sail to a desired destination, a ship's captain will have plotted a course by taking into account winds, current, and distance, as well as the capacity of the crew, and the fitness and weight of the vessel. While hoping for "fair sailing," the captain and crew will inevitably have to make midcourse corrections based on circumstances that arise as a result of changes in the weather or perhaps unforeseen problems with the vessel. Course corrections are more likely on longer voyages that require intermediate stops before reaching the final destination. The magnitude of the corrections will depend on (1) the nature of the problem that arises, (2) the point in the voyage at which a problem or condition is detected, (3) the skills of the captain and crew, and (4) the capabilities of the vessel. All of the relevant events of the trip will be recorded in the *ship's log,* which will serve as a key source for insights that will serve to enhance performance on subsequent voyages.

The navigational metaphor of evaluation is appropriate for health promotion practitioners because the best "evidence" of their performance will come from their ability to describe current program status accurately, in light of their program goals and objectives, and taking into account emerging conditions and events.

Earlier, we mentioned that "skills" can be important enabling factors. The following example from our own experience illustrates both the practical and the ethical importance of making a commitment to evaluation. Several years ago, a group of physicians wanted us to help teach senior citizens with hypertension how to take one another's blood pressure. The physicians hoped that teaching the seniors those skills would result in a decrease in the number of unnecessary office visits. Prior to launching the program, we decided to do a small pilot study. A group of seniors were randomly assigned to either an intervention group or a control group. Intervention subjects were taught how to use the sphygmomanometer and stethoscope on one another and to record their readings. We had experienced previous success using similar methods with junior-high students. As a part of the formative aspect of our evaluation plan, we had scheduled one site visit per week. During the first visit, the signs of impending disaster were already apparent. Although most of the participants reported that they felt pleased and empowered with their new ability, several were frustrated and indicated that the program made them "downright angry" because it reminded them of their shortcomings.

The causes for the unhappiness were multiple. Some had arthritis severe enough to prohibit them from squeezing the bulb on the sphygmomanometer. Others had visual impairments that hindered their ability to read the measurements. Feedback was immediate and had a discouraging effect. This situation provides us with a clear-cut example of why evaluation is important. Evaluation of the pilot project uncovered flaws in the analysis that, left unchecked, could lead to health impairment rather than health improvement!

Our commitment to monitoring program activities, like the captain and crew looking for changes in weather or currents, enabled us to detect a problem and make the necessary changes to correct it. The complexity of human behavior, combined with the complexity of the social forces and conditions that influence health, make it virtually impossible to plan a program that will not require adjustments along the way.

The Framework for Program Evaluation, developed by the Centers for Disease Control and Prevention,[7] offers practitioners a comprehensive set of principles to guide them in their evaluation efforts. Figure 4.8 depicts program evaluation as a cycle consisting of six, interdependent steps, wherein the earlier steps provide the foundation for subsequent steps. As we walk through the six steps, you will see the how key elements covered in previous chapters are integral to the overall process.

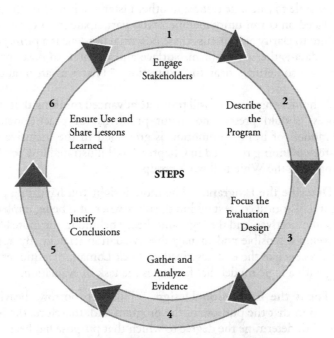

FIGURE 4.8 Steps in Program Evaluation

Step 1: Engage Stakeholders.   Stakeholders are individuals (1) who are involved in development and implementation of the program (e.g., program sponsors or funders, administrators, coalition partners, community participants, local media, and staff) or (2) who are served or affected by the program (e.g., community residents, clients or students, neighborhood organizations, and advocacy groups). The emphasis on *participation* in Chapter 3 reinforces the critical importance of the early participation, or engagement, of stakeholders in all aspects of evaluation.

Here are two practical examples of stakeholder engagement, specific to the task of evaluation. First, all stakeholders, but especially administrators and those responsible for funding, should be consulted in those deliberations that will determine what constitutes realistic and acceptable program outcomes. Their input, combined with their understanding of the context in which the program will be implemented, will increase the probability that the desired outcomes will be realistic and that expectations will be shared from the outset.

A second example of stakeholder engagement reflects the reality that data and information used in the evaluation process come from a variety of sources. To varying degrees, gathering that information will inevitably require an investment of time and effort, and frequently it will involve effort put forth by those other than program staff. In some instances, it may be the effort made by coalition members in their search of relevant databases that will make it possible to calculate trends; in other instances, it may be the response burden placed on community members who participate in interviews or surveys. Failure to clarify and discuss these potential burdens is a primary reason why, after data-gathering problems surface and threaten to delay or disrupt programs, we sometimes hear the expression, "That was an unanticipated problem!"

Stakeholder engagement will promote advanced thinking that is shared. The process should present no major problems for practitioners whose "mental model" of health promotion is grounded in the inclusive ethic of participatory planning reflected in Chapter 3 and illustrated in Dick Loman's interaction with the Whitehall work group.

Step 2: Describe the Program.   The more insight you have on a program, its social and historical context within the place where it is being implemented, its goals and objectives, and the logic and theory behind it, the more likely you are to develop a sensible and manageable evaluation strategy. By applying a planning process like the one described by Dick Loman, practitioners will be operating with a logic model that facilitates the task of evaluation.

Step 3: Focus the Evaluation Design.   This step borrows heavily from the first step in that the purpose of the program and, therefore, the information needed to determine the degree to which that purpose has been reached, is understood and agreed upon by stakeholders. By attending to this step, practitioners seek clarification and insights into the following questions:

- What is the primary purpose(s) for conducting the evaluation (to develop new knowledge, modify practices, influence policy change, justify political support, or demonstrate accountability)?
- Given the time and resource limitations, what procedures are most likely to yield accurate and reliable information?
- Who (persons or groups) will receive evaluation results or benefit from being part of the evaluation?
- How will the findings be applied?

Step 4: Gather and Analyze Evidence.   In this book, we have placed great emphasis on the notion that evaluation and sound planning are interdependent processes. Accordingly, throughout the planning process, practitioners should be on the lookout for dimensions of evidence: *indicators of evidence* and *sources of evidence.* An indicator of evidence is a marker that provides a direct or indirect measure or record of the degree to which an event of interest has or has not occurred.

Suppose you were part of the community group working on a youth tobacco-control program that included a collaborative component with local law enforcement authorities to redress the well-documented reality that existing sales-to-minors laws were not being enforced. Several potential *indicators of evidence* could be linked to the enforcement of such laws. Note how the following examples represent a graduating sequence of indicators that lead to the goal of enforcement:

1. Meeting with law enforcement, business leaders, and the Chamber of Commerce to verify the problem
2. Identifying barriers to enforcement
3. Developing strategies to address priority barriers
4. Securing resources to implement those strategies
5. Documenting the implementation and impact of those strategies (e.g., training programs for law enforcement officers and managers of retail outlets)
6. Documenting enforcement

For examples 1 and 5, *the source of evidence* is likely to come from logs or activity forms. Documented group assessments are the likely sources for examples 2 and 4 (barriers and strategies). Narratives of budget records would be the likely source for example 4 (evidence for securing resources). Evidence for example 6 (the presence or absence of enforcement) could come from three sources: direct observation, personal interviews, or surveys.

Step 5: Justify Conclusions. Let's return to the hypothetical youth tobacco-control program mentioned in the previous step. Suppose a county commissioner, known to be supportive of public health, comes up to the health promotion practitioner managing that program and asks the following question: Is the program working? Which of the three answers below would be *least* useful to the commissioner?

- We got off to a slow start with budget problems but our coalition has been very helpful in turning that around. We're running about six months behind, but we have hired two new part-time staff members and can document good progress, especially on our media campaign and on the retail stores outreach program.
- I'm really enthusiastic about it and think it is going real well.
- We've completed the teacher training component; it will be in place in all the elementary schools next year. Our coalition has also developed a first draft of the policy strategy for indoor clean air.

Although heartfelt and well intended, the second response is without meaningful information or substance. At best, it may prompt a second question probing for examples, but officials like the commissioner are busy people and follow-up queries may not be forthcoming. The first and third responses communicate substance. In the first example, note how the identification of a problem (slow start) is framed around specific actions to move forward. The third example provides simple, but tangible examples of progress.

Step 6: Ensure Use and Share Lessons Learned. Programs are evaluated to provide documentation about (1) how the program is working and (2) how well its goals and objectives are being met. Documentation has value only to the extent that it is used. In the earlier example of the hypertension self-care program for senior citizens, the evaluation component enabled program staff to detect potential negative effects early on.

Making necessary program adjustments will constitute a practitioner's most frequent and routine use of program evaluation information. However, that same information should be regularly communicated to all stakeholders, especially those participants or community members targeted by the program.

When routinely apprised of program status, stakeholders (including administrators and those who "invest" in the program) will be more likely to maintain their interest, support, and commitment. This is true even when a program is falling short of its goals, so long as evidence explaining the situation is clearly communicated and corrective strategies are explained. Failure to keep stakeholders informed can be interpreted as a manifestation of disinterest in their feedback or a lack of trust in their views.

These steps remind us that we need evidence to determine how our programs are working, and that we need to use the evidence as the primary basis to (1) enhance the quality of those programs and (2) keep stakeholders up-to-date about program status and progress.

Finding Evaluation Evidence: An Example

The following case provides a hypothetical example of how evaluation "evidence" is used in a practical setting. The Longview metropolitan area has a population of 233,013, 26.1 percent of whom are youths aged 5–17 years. The 1997 State Annual Health Report indicated that one out of every 5.3 deaths in the state was tobacco-related and that tobacco accounted for $2.6 billion in hospital costs. The 1998 State Youth Tobacco Survey (SYTS), coordinated by the state health department, oversampled the community of Longview. Specifically, anonymous questionnaires were sent to 2300 high school students. Results from that survey indicated that 40 percent of Longview high school students used cigarettes at least once in the previous 30 days. That rate was nine percentage points above the statewide average.

In a 1999 survey conducted jointly by the Longview Health Department and Longview School District, 13.5 percent of sixth-grade students answered "yes" to the following question: "Have you used cigarettes in the last 30 days?" The same survey revealed that 24 percent of male seventh-graders reported using cigarettes or smokeless tobacco at least once in the previous 30 days. In early 2000, concerned citizens in Longview joined forces with local public health and school officials to form the Healthy Longview Children Coalition (HLCC). The HLCC, consisting of 25 stakeholders, declared that, to make Longview a healthy place to raise children, one of its first priorities was to address the problem of tobacco and health. *Observing that the survey data indicated that tobacco use intensifies as teens move through school, the HLCC concluded that tobacco prevention efforts targeted at middle school and high school youth may be "too late."*

In September 2000, the coalition received grant funding from a large private health foundation. A planning process, based on a community assessment carried out by the coalition, developed the primary intervention goal of minimizing the onset of tobacco use by (1) reducing the accessibility and availability of tobacco to minors and (2) increasing the number of restaurants, businesses, and workplaces that voluntarily adopted a 100 percent smoke-free policy. Funding for years 3 and 4 would be contingent upon evidence of progress in years 1 and 2.

Based on the intervention priorities, the following tactics were deemed the most promising to help the coalition achieve its goal of reducing tobacco use among youth:

- Modifying the selling practices of merchants
- Increasing enforcement of existing laws
- Restricting smoking in public places

TABLE 4.3   Selected Baseline and Follow-up Indicators

Indicator	Baseline 1998–1999	Follow-up 2001
Percentage of sixth-grade students who used tobacco in the last 30 days	11.2%	11%
Percentage of current smokers (middle school) who buy cigarettes at gas stations or convenience stores	63%	21%
Percentage of current smokers (middle school) who purchased cigarettes but were not asked to show proof of age	72%	34%
Number of restaurants that are entirely smoke-free	46% (17/37)	62% (27/37)
Number of Longview merchants (clerks) who ask for verification of age before selling cigarettes	62% (34/55)	91% (51/55)
Longview Merchants Association: sponsor minors access training	No	Yes
Longview minor league baseball team: adopt a policy prohibiting tobacco sponsorship and advertising	No	Under negotiation
Longview Board of Education: a uniform ban on tobacco use for students, teachers, and staff, not only on school grounds but at all school-related functions	No	On board agenda
Enforcement-related activities reported by the LPD:		
☐ Inspections for signs?	No	Yes
☐ Conduct periodic compliance checks?	Yes	Yes
☐ Issue citations?	No	Yes
☐ Issue awards/letters for compliance?	No	Yes
☐ Use volunteers in tobacco enforcement?	No	Yes

Eighteen months after the grant had been awarded (in March 2002), Chris Meanswell, the program coordinator, was asked to brief the HLCC stakeholders on the progress of the program prior to their meeting with the mayor and City Council. Chris relied on two sources of information in preparing his briefing: a table comparing selected indicators before and after receipt of the grant and implementation of the program (Table 4.3) and a log of program activities (Table 4.4).

Imagine that you are one of the stakeholders. Given the program goals, would this kind of information help you form an opinion on how well the program is progressing? Would the evidence in these two tables make you more or less inclined to support other health promotions planned in a similar fashion? How difficult would it be to assemble this kind of information?

TABLE 4.4   HLCC Quarterly Progress Log: Verified Changes in the Longview Community and Systems Environment Related to Tobacco-Use Prevention

Verified Events (New or Modified Programs, Policies, or Practices)	Date
1. HLCC issues report cards to registered voters grading elected officials' tobacco-related voting record	May 13, 2001
2. Schools teach media literacy using tobacco advertising as a case example	May 18, 2001
3. Rails to Trails Consortium initiates a monthly campaign to collect cigarette butts (and other litter) in parks, along roadsides, and in other public places	June 4, 2001
4. HLCC and R-T Consortium hold a joint press conference after cigarette cleanup day to highlight the environmental damage done by tobacco products	June 4, 2001
5. Teen advisory board established to guide the HLCC tobacco prevention initiative	July 14, 2001
6. Bars, restaurants, and grocery stores agree not to distribute free matches to youth	July 22, 2001
7. Monthly reports are circulated to small business owners that summarize all recent citations and fines issued for selling tobacco to minors	August 15, 2001
8. Merchants raise prices on matches and lighters	November 2, 2001
9. Paid community mobilizers start working for the HLCC initiative	December 15, 2001
10. Longview Town Cinema holds a free screening of *The Insider*	February 12, 2001
11. School sports teams require participants to sign a no-smoking pact	February 18, 2001
12. Longview city government, schools, and community organizations participate in the Great American Smokeout	April 7, 2001
13. Schools and youth-serving organizations display posters from the "Celebrities Against Smoking" series	April 15, 2001
14. Longview minor league baseball team adopts and is enforcing a policy prohibiting tobacco sponsorship and advertising	May 4, 2002
15. Longview School Board announces the passage of a uniform ban on tobacco use for students, teachers, and staff, not only on school grounds, but at all school-related functions	May 15, 2002
16. Longview Chamber of Commerce and Rotary Club jointly endorse "Smoke-Free Seal of Health" signs for merchants who do not sell tobacco to minors	May 27, 2002

(continued)

TABLE 4.4 *continued*

Verified Events (New or Modified Programs, Policies, or Practices)	Date
17. Longview Police Department recruits and trains a Youth Tobacco Sting Unit to enforce tobacco access restrictions	May 30, 2002
18. Longview art museum holds first annual "You Smoke, You Choke" artwork contest	June 2, 2002
19. Longview Merchants Association sponsors minors' tobacco access training	June 5, 2002
20. Longview Police Department instructs patrol officers to inspect for the presence of signs about tobacco age restrictions	July 2, 2002
21. Longview Police Department instructs patrol officers to issue citations for illegal tobacco sales	July 2, 2002
22. Longview Police Department issues awards/letters for merchants who consistently comply with tobacco laws	July 2, 2002
23. Longview HMO sponsors weekly smoking-cessation classes	September 9, 2002
24. Case managers are assigned to work with pregnant and parenting teens who smoke	October 13, 2002

SUMMARY

How often we have heard the story of caring practitioners—with virtually no resources available to obtain baseline data or evaluations—who use their experience and knowledge of local circumstances to create innovative programs, after which local observers express the strong sentiment and belief that the program "worked" or "made a difference." However, when the time inevitably comes to demonstrate the effect of such programs, the practitioner discovers that sentiment is no match for documented evidence.

We suspect that in many of these instances, there probably are genuine effects, most of which unfortunately go undetected. If practitioners adopt an analytical planning approach like the one described in this chapter, they will automatically build in the essential ingredients required to make their program efforts amenable to evaluation. By identifying high-priority problems and the behavioral and environmental risks associated with those problems, by framing measurable objectives and creating specific tactics to achieve those objectives, and by being mindful of the core steps of program evaluation, you put into place the markers for evaluation. Furthermore, by taking this kind of accountable approach, practitioners will find, just as Rachel Warren discovered, that stakeholders will become engaged and more likely to understand and support your efforts.

ENDNOTES

1. In this context, by "environmental factors" we primarily mean the social conditions that can have a direct or indirect influence on either a health behavior or a specific health problem. For example, these factors include organizational or social policies (e.g., laws pertaining to the sale of tobacco to youth, speed limits, indoor clear air acts, health insurance regulations, standards for screening and immunization). In some instances, the physical environment may be especially relevant, as in the case of poor road conditions, insufficient lighting in a building, standing water that breeds mosquitoes, lead paint, and dust.

2. Green LW, Kreuter MW. *Health Promotion Planning: An Educational and Ecological Approach,* 3rd ed. Menlo Park, CA: Mayfield Publishing; 1999. To date, there have been more than 900 published accounts of the model. See http://www.lgreen.net/bibliog.htm or http://www.ihpr.ubc.ca/index_ihpr.htm.

3. The basic assumption underlying Stages of Change theory is that behavior change can be best understood as a series of steps or stages of transition from resistance to taking a given action to taking and repeating that action. For a good review of the theory, we suggest Prochaska JO, DiClemente CC, Norcross JC. In search of how people change: applications to addictive behaviors. *Am Psychologist.* 1992;47:1102–1114.

4. The primary difference between stating objectives for behaviors and for environmental factors is that the *who* question is usually not included in stating the environmental objective.

5. Donna Cross, Peter Howatt, Steve Jones, Mark Stevenson, and Margaret Hall and their colleagues at the Western Australian Centre of Health Promotion Research at Curtin University in Perth, Australia, gave us permission to use their adaptation of the Precede–Proceed model they have employed to guide their research and development of the Child Pedestrian Injury Prevention Project in Western Australia. Howatt P, Jones S, Hall M, Cross D, Stevenson M. The PRECEDE-PROCEED model: Application to planning a child pedestrian injury prevention program. *Injury Prev.* 1997;3(6):282–287.

6. Romer D, Black M, Ricardo I, Feigelman S, Daljee L, Galbraith J, et al. Social influences of youth at risk for HIV exposure. *Am J Public Health.* 1994; 84(6):977–985.

7. We are grateful to Bobby Milstein, Goldie MacDonald, and Michael Schooley of the CDC for sharing their ideas and expertise in developing the evaluation section of this chapter. The CDC Program Evaluation Framework can be found in Centers for Disease Control and Prevention, *Framework Program Evaluation in Public Health. MMWR.* 1999; 40(No. RR-11). Also see www.cdc.gov/eval/framework.htm.

CHAPTER 5

Theory Applied

Case Story
THE OLD HORSE

His granddaughter called him Lao Ma ("old horse") because one of her favorite pastimes was to climb up on his back and ride him around the house. In addition to being an "old horse," he was also known as Dr. Yu Mei, director of the Ministry of Public Health (MOPH) for Zhejiang Province in the People's Republic of China. Dr. Yu was a highly respected public health official in China who had distinguished himself through his pioneering public health work. In 1980, he received international recognition when the World Health Organization (WHO) honored him with a distinguished service medal for his accomplishments in tuberculosis (TB) control. Dr. Yu was an advocate of health education because it had been an essential part of his TB prevention and control efforts.

The literal English translation of the Chinese expression for the term *health education* is "health propaganda." This definition fits the Chinese tradition of public campaigns that used banners, posters, pamphlets, and community lectures to communicate health messages. The central government had established an entity called the National Patriotic Health Campaign Committee (NPHCC) to provide national health education leadership; virtually all communities in China have a local NPHCC.

Like many of his Chinese public health colleagues, Dr. Yu was well aware that his country was experiencing a health transition: better control of communicable and infectious diseases meant that more people would survive to adulthood, which in turn meant that more people would be at risk for chronic health problems such as heart disease, stroke, and cancers. Dr. Yu knew that the disturbing smoking trends in China made this pattern of transition more problematic. Virtually all of the surveys on tobacco use showed that nearly 70 percent of men in China smoked. And, although the surveys indicated that few women in China were smokers, an increase in smoking among younger women was occurring, especially in the larger cities. Dr. Yu was also aware that as China continued to move ahead as a market-driven economy, its health profile would surely begin to reflect those of some other market economies, including both the positive and negative effects of market forces.

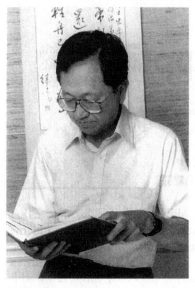

Dr. Yu Mei

Because of his expertise in tuberculosis prevention, Dr. Yu was a frequent consultant to WHO in Geneva. Through his contact with WHO, he became aware of the health education and health promotion innovations that were emerging in areas of public health other than TB; he viewed the cardiovascular risk-reduction programs in Europe, Scandinavia, Canada, Australia, and the United States with keen interest. These programs were more complex and went beyond the traditional Chinese approach to health education. Dr. Yu was eager to experiment with these Western methods to see if they could be adapted as part of the prevention strategy in his health ministry.

Dr. Yu was especially interested in the community intervention work being carried out by Dr. Pekka Puska and his co-workers in Finland. As Dr. Yu developed long-range prevention plans for his province, he frequently sought the counsel of Dr. Puska.

Dr. Li Fang (pronounced "Lee Fong") had completed her medical training at Shanghai Medical University and then stayed on for an additional year of studies in public health. Her dream of returning to her home province to practice public health was realized in January when she accepted an offer from Dr. Yu to become the health education coordinator for the Zhejiang Province MOPH.

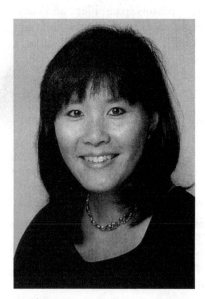

Dr. Li Fang

In some regions of China, it is customary for friends and co-workers, especially when speaking informally, to refer to younger persons by placing the word *xiao* (pronounced "shao") before their names. So, outside of formal circles, with courtesy and respect, Dr. Li Fang was called Xiao Fang. In Xiao Fang, Dr. Yu was hopeful that he had found the person who could take a leadership role in implementing a new vision of health education and health promotion in Zhejiang Province.

During her first six months on the job, Xiao Fang spent the majority of her time working alongside co-workers from other units of the MOPH as a part of the MOPH planning team. Their task was to prepare the Provincial Health Plan for the Year 2010, modeled in part after the WHO *Health for All by the Year 2000* documents and *Healthy People 2010,* a health promotion/ disease prevention planning document developed in the United States.

Xiao Fang and her colleagues pored through mounds of data and reports. They looked at patterns and trends of health problems and risk factors, then compared those patterns with the usual social, economic, educational, and employment variables. As they began to identify high-priority problems and formulate health objectives, they could not deny the magnitude of the problem of tobacco consumption. Data on smoking and health in China were shocking: World Bank studies showed that tobacco was causing about 500,000 deaths per year in China, half of which were attributable to chronic lung disease. Left unchecked, the rate of tobacco consumption among men (70 percent) would lead to an epidemic of unnecessary chronic diseases; it would cause premature death and disability that would, by 2020 or 2030, have the joint effect of diminishing the workforce and crippling the Chinese system of health. The chilling reality about this effect was not whether—but precisely when—it would occur.

In May, after members of the MOPH advisory council had reviewed a working draft of the Provincial Health Plan for the Year 2010, Dr. Yu announced that tobacco-use prevention and control would be one of the top health priorities for the MOPH. He also announced that he was assigning Xiao Fang to take the lead in developing an anti-tobacco demonstration project for one of the communities within the province. He needed to show that a planned tobacco-use prevention and control program was feasible and could be effective. Once Dr. Yu was able to show effectiveness and feasibility, dissemination throughout the province, and perhaps to the rest of China, would follow.

Dr. Yu informed Xiao Fang that he would make arrangements for her to participate in the two-week community-intervention training course held each year by Dr. Puska and his colleagues in early July at Joensuu, North Karelia, Finland. The announcement for the training course indicated that it would include several experts who had developed tobacco-use control programs in other countries; the timing couldn't have been better. Xiao Fang's excitement about the trip was tempered by the reality that she was undertaking a large responsibility and had much to accomplish before leaving for Finland.

The Eastern District of the city of Hangzhou was chosen as the demonstration site. Xiao Fang's first step was to assemble a planning group, aptly named the No-Smoking Team. First, she got the support and participation of the local Patriotic Health Campaign Committee. Next, she successfully recruited key representatives from hospitals, schools, businesses, volunteer cancer agencies, and the media. With the support and counsel of Dr. Yu, the

No-Smoking Team was able to secure the participation of two of the Eastern District's key political figures. The planning process was under way.

* * *

In July, northern Finland is the land of the midnight sun. Xiao Fang was taken by the fact that the sun never seemed to set; it turned out to be quite appropriate, though, because she was far more interested in exploring new ideas than in sleeping! She had read most of the literature published on the cardiovascular community-intervention trials and had a good general understanding of the process. What she wanted out of the training was more detail, especially about the methods and the thinking that led to those methods. She framed all of her questions in terms of the tobacco-use prevention and control task she and her co-workers in the Eastern District of Hangzhou had in front of them. New information and interesting ideas were everywhere, but two concepts stood out for Xiao Fang.

The first had to do with school health education. Xiao Fang and members of the No-Smoking Team had recognized that schools were likely to play a major role in whatever program emerged. In the training, she learned that with thoughtful planning schools could serve as an effective means to reach and engage the support of parents. One of the visiting faculty members, Dr. Cheryl Perry from Minnesota, presented evidence from her work in Minnesota and other American programs that school-based approaches could have an influence upon specific health habits of parents.

The second important concept was a theory that suggested that individual human health behavior changes in accordance to the extent to which an individual is more or less ready to change. Appropriately called the Stages of Change model, this theory sets forth the proposition that behavior change is not a single event, but rather a series of events that depend upon an individual's readiness to change. According to this theory, there are five different levels of readiness to make and sustain changes. The names of the stages are almost self-explanatory. For example, the stage in which a person is furthest from attempting a change is called the precontemplation stage; the next stage is contemplation; then comes the ready for action or decision stage, followed by the action stage. The final stage is called maintenance.

As Xiao Fang thought more about this theory, it seemed clear that there were real possibilities for its application in the tobacco-use prevention and control program she and her colleagues were planning. She thought to herself, "If a large number of men in the Eastern District are not in the ready for action stage, a large campaign on smoking cessation may not be a good investment of time and effort."

She also learned that numerous studies in the United States had used standardized questions in surveys to determine the distribution of levels of readiness to change within populations. Thus, not only was it possible to measure these stages of change in a population of smokers, but it was also possible to detect whether changes occur in the stages over time. Dr. Yu was unambiguous about the issue of evaluation; he had made repeated references to his desire to see some evidence of program effects.

Xiao Fang had much to share with her colleagues back in Hangzhou.

* * *

Twenty people were seated around the long table, which was dotted with cups containing loose ground tea, large Thermos jugs full of piping hot water, and small bowls of fresh fruit. Senior staff from the Zhejiang Province MOPH were joined by members of the No-Smoking Team. No one was more eager to hear Xiao Fang's debriefing report than Dr. Yu.

She began with a few slides of the Joensuu countryside. "This is a picture of our hotel at 12 noon; this is our hotel at 3 a.m. As you can see, no difference!" The ensuing chuckle was polite.

After providing a brief summary of the content covered in the training program, Xiao Fang began to describe how the No-Smoking Team members could strengthen their school health approach by adding a specific component designed to reach parents. She then shifted attention to the possible application of Stages of Change theory. She explained how, by incorporating just a few questions into their baseline survey, the public health workers could realize two benefits: (1) some valuable information to help them plan their intervention and (2) data showing whether their program caused a shift in the population of men's readiness to quit smoking.

Dr. Yu sat back and observed the questions and discussion that Xiao Fang's report had stimulated. After a most animated and lively exchange, consensus was reached that translation of the Stages of Change questions into Chinese would not compromise the construct being measured. Dr. Yu said little.

* * *

Baseline surveys were initiated in the middle of August. By October, the No-Smoking Team had the results from the Stages of Change measurements. Approximately 68 percent of the men and 7 percent of the women sampled were regular smokers. Of the men who smoked, 72 percent fell into the precontemplation category—meaning that they had yet to consider quitting. (Another American term Xiao Fang had learned for this stage was the word "denial.") The survey also showed that among youths aged 13 to 15, 34 percent of boys and 4 percent of girls reported that they smoked at least occasionally.

Liu Baoyi had been assigned to take the lead in preparing the intervention plan. He had been a part of the health education team for the MOPH's successful tuberculosis-control program. A popular and well-respected figure in the Eastern District, Liu Baoyi was known more for his accomplishments as the premier soccer coach for young people in the community than for his work with the MOPH.

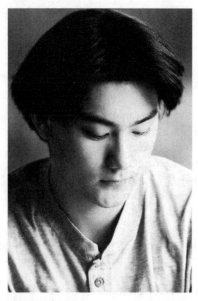

Liu Baoyi

After getting comments on a first draft of the plan, Liu Baoyi presented the final proposed strategy to the No-Smoking Team on September 1. He explained that they would take a comprehensive approach involving the local cancer society, businesses, and media, as well as the local Patriotic Health Campaign Committee. The focal point for the program was to be the Eastern District school system. It included four primary components:

• A health curriculum that placed emphasis on teaching children about the harmful effects of smoking and was variably tailored for students in grades 2 through 6

• A coordinated media campaign wherein the radio, television, and newspapers featured stories and information about the health effects of tobacco

• Smoking-cessation self-help clinics that were promoted and made accessible through the local volunteer cancer organization

• A planned effort by local political officials advocating the implementation of policies that promoted smoke-free areas in public places and businesses

Next, Liu Baoyi explained that planning had been influenced by two key points: (1) timing and (2) the application of the Stages of Change theory within the context of traditional Chinese cultural beliefs.

He gave a brief review of the analysis of smoking prevalence data and an overview of the Stages of Change theory. He then concluded by pointing out that the baseline data clearly showed that the majority of male smokers were in the precontemplative stage of change.[1]

Liu Baoyi announced, "Here is our strategy to reach them: May 31 is World No-Tobacco Day and June 1 is Children's Day.[2] Since we know that a large majority of fathers are smokers who are precontemplatives, we have arranged for all the children to bring home a letter to their fathers the day before World No-Tobacco Day. The letter will read:

Dear Father:

This letter comes from the bottom of my heart.

I have been learning about the harm of smoking in school and my heart is heavy. Science shows us that smoking can cause lung cancer and heart disease and cause death before people get old. Also, the smoke from others can harm those who do not smoke.

It worries me to see you smoke.

As I grow up, I will need your love and wisdom to help me. Tomorrow is "World No-Tobacco Day"; won't you please consider giving up smoking?

The day after tomorrow is "Children's Day." The best present I can get is not a toy but a promise that you will try to stop smoking.

I love you, Father.

(Signed by the child)

Liu Baoyi continued, "The school curriculum and all the media events will point to the importance of No-Tobacco Day and Children's Day. We will work with local political leaders to promote the adoption of no-smoking policies in schools, other public buildings, and voluntarily in businesses. The local volunteer cancer organization will make it known to everyone that free smoking-cessation clinics, at convenient hours, will be available for the entire month of June."

*   *   *

The National Chronic Disease Prevention Meeting was held in Tianjin, about 50 kilometers north of Beijing. Dr. Yu sat in the back of the auditorium. Although his demeanor was reserved on the outside, he was beaming on the inside as Xiao Fang came to her closing remarks:

Again, there were 10,500 students (in grades 2 through 6) in the intervention group and 9987 students in the reference group. Although the knowledge scores were similar for the two groups at baseline, students in the intervention group had significantly higher knowledge scores (40 percent) at follow-up.

Smoking rates of fathers in both groups were the same at baseline (68 percent); that translated into 6843 smokers in the intervention population. The stages-of-change data were also approximately the same—at baseline, 74 percent of smokers in the intervention group were precontemplatives, and the figure was 76 percent for smokers in the reference population. At follow-up, 61 percent of the precontemplatives in the intervention group reported a shift in stage to "contemplation" or "ready for action"; there was no significant shift among fathers in the reference group.

Finally, the data on smoking cessation were most encouraging. Self-reported data indicated that 90 percent of the 6843 had quit for 10 days, 64 percent were still not smoking at 20 days, 30 percent at 60 days, and 11 percent at 210 days. For men in the reference population, only 2 percent reported a quit attempt in the first 10 days, and after 210 days the overall quit rate was 0.2 percent.

These findings suggest to us that a carefully planned, comprehensive tobacco-use prevention program that uses a school-based focus can be effective not only in improving the health knowledge of children, but also in predisposing previously unmotivated adults to quit smoking or at least to be more amenable to trying, and in encouraging other adults who were somewhat motivated to actually try to quit.

Let me close with this epidemiological extrapolation: There are currently about 250 million smokers in China. If our program were implemented throughout the country and similar outcomes were attained, the result would be that 27 million smokers would have quit for 210 days. That is a dream we would very much like to pursue. Thank you.

The old horse smiled.

Case Analysis

The success of Li Fang's smoking-control efforts in China illustrates how a practitioner's understanding of theory can be directly applied to influence a health promotion program. We know that her thoughts about intervention were filtered through the lens of Stages of Change theory, and that those thoughts were influential in shaping the program that eventually emerged. We suspect that the thought processes of Li Fang and her co-workers probably went something like this:

Question: What portion of all smokers are in the precontemplation stage?
Answer: Our survey data tell us that a great majority of those who smoke are in the precontemplation stage.
Action: Add Stages of Change questions to our baseline survey.
Question: What does that tell us?
Answer: Three ideas stand out: (1) if we use methods aimed at smokers that emphasize the health hazards of smoking or that implore smokers to join cessation clinics, such methods won't have much of an effect on smokers who are precontemplative; (2) it would be unrealistic for us to set quitting as the immediate goal; and (3) precontemplatives are resistant to cognitive messages that emphasize the detrimental health effects of tobacco. They are more likely to respond to affective approaches that appeal to more

ultimate values than the value they hold for their own immediate
health.

Actions: Our health problem is clear: tobacco causes unnecessary death
and disability. Our program goal is also clear: to improve health by
reducing the consumption of tobacco. Theory suggests that since
behavior changes in stages, a prudent and scientifically sound first
step would be to design and employ tactics that have a high probability of enhancing smokers' readiness to quit. One approach
might be to try to move smokers from the precontemplation stage
to the contemplation stage by appealing to a traditional Chinese
value: As elders hold a position of respect and honor in Chinese
culture, it is their duty to pass their wisdom on to children. A possible message from children to their fathers might be, "Please don't
do something that might compromise your ability to give me your
wisdom and direction in the future."

From the perspective of health promotion practice, using theory is a lot
like using a road map. First, you have to have a good idea about where you're
going. Just as road maps can't help you if you don't know your destination, so
theories have little practical value if you don't have a good grasp of the problem or issue you are trying to resolve. Most of the theories applied in health
promotion programs are useful because they map out the process of how
individuals, organizations, and communities change.

By understanding these processes, you can determine which roads are
most likely to lead you to the desired outcomes. Without a road map, you will
be forced to do a lot of guessing about which road to take, an effort that is
likely to use up precious time and fuel. Similarly, inefficiency results when
you try to frame interventions without applying theory. Thus, using theories
to guide interventions will increase your chances of meeting program objectives and doing so in the most efficient way possible.

The remainder of this chapter is divided into two sections. The first section provides an introductory discussion of theory, including a few ideas to
help practitioners in the process of deciding which theories are most applicable to the specific circumstances they face. In the second section, we review
several theories that are commonly applied by practitioners and provide examples of how elements of those theories inform the decisions that practitioners make about interventions.

THEORY: A PRIMER

Consider this definition of theory: "a set of interrelated concepts, definitions,
and propositions that present a systematic view of events or situations by
specifying relationships among variables to explain or predict the events or

situations."[3] Whew! How does this academic definition translate into every-day actions?

Whether in our routine day-to-day tasks or our professional lives, our every action is grounded in some sort of "theory." In fact, we are hard-pressed to think of any conscious actions you might take in absence of some theory.

For example, consider the routine that many of us follow when arriving home after dark. We open the door, reach inside, and flip the light switch with the expectation that the lights will turn on. Whether consciously or not, our expectation is grounded in our belief that when we flip the switch, sufficient electrical current will flow to the light bulb socket and, assuming the light bulb is functional and properly affixed to the socket, the lights will go on.

Borrowing from the terms used in the definition cited previously, we put together a set of interrelated concepts and propositions (switches, electrical current, light bulbs), which in turn give us a systematic view of events that help specify relationships among variables. (Flipping the switch activates electrical current and starts a causal chain of events, assuming that all parts of the system are functional.) These thought processes serve as the basis for predicting an event (the lights will go on!). Of course, most of us become cognizant that we hold a "theory of house lighting" only when we flip the switch and nothing happens. The distress and accompanying level of frustration we experience will in large part be determined by the steps we take to solve that problem—those with a faulty theory are likely to take more time and experience more frustration than those who act on a sound theory.

Activists and scholars from Saul Alinsky and Paulo Freire to Meredith Minkler have consistently reminded practitioners to pay attention to the principle of participation and the process of respectfully engaging the community.[4] In Chapter 3, we discussed these important concepts not as theories per se but, as the title of this book implies, as critical community health promotion ideas that work. As you proceed with the remainder of this chapter, you will note that it emphasizes theories that explain behavior and the precursors to behavior. Accordingly, we urge you to carefully examine this sampling of theories within the context of the community settings where they are inevitably played out.

Once the focus of the health promotion program (i.e., the behavioral or environmental problem and the demographic, social, and economic context of that problem) has been clearly defined and agreed upon, practitioners may find it helpful to seek insights by finding the answers to three simple questions:

1. Is the theory relevant to my problem?

2. How does the theory help me understand targets for change?

3. How does the theory help in the selection or development of an intervention method or tactic?

Is the Theory Relevant to My Problem?

With detailed information about the kinds of behavioral and environmental factors that contribute to the problem, you can determine which theories, if any, provide a good explanation or understanding of the problem you've selected. For example, are those people who are affected by the problem actually aware of the problem? Do they think it is a risk for them? Do they have the skills and motivation to take preventive action? Are solutions to the problem affordable and accessible? What kind of social pressures or social support would they experience for or against action? Is the community ready to support change? Depending upon the nature of the problem, some theories may be more useful than others. For many problems, especially complex ones, no single theory will fully address the problem, and it will be necessary to consider and combine multiple theories or parts of multiple theories.

How Does the Theory Help Me Understand Targets for Change?

Most theories propose a set of conditions or relationships under which changes are most likely to occur. In doing so, they implicitly identify targets for change. For example, if having a strong social support system is one of the key concepts in a particular theory of behavior change, that theory might predict that people with less social support would be less likely to make behavioral changes. Social support, then, is identified as one possible target for change. It follows that for this particular theory, effective programs designed to enhance social support should increase the likelihood of achieving the desired outcome.

How Does the Theory Help in the Selection or Development of an Intervention Method or Tactic?

Once theory leads us to the best targets for health promotion programs, specific strategies must be developed to address those targets. Some theories go beyond explaining behavior, suggesting types of support or intervention to achieve or increase the likelihood of change. As in the previous example, if lack of social support was the cause of the problem, it follows that we would need to find ways to enhance social support. While this goal can be accomplished in many ways (e.g., working with other family members, setting up a support group or telephone hotline, establishing an online computer user group), the challenge is selecting those tactics that will best address the problem as it exists in the population of interest. Unfortunately, there are no quick and easy ways to do so. Reading journal articles about other programs that have addressed the same problem can help you generate ideas, as can conversations with other practitioners and community members. Most importantly, you should pretest whatever tactics you decide are best with the members of the target population. Their evaluation of the appropriateness and usefulness of a program is critical.

THEORY SUMMARIES

Keeping in mind the spirit of the three questions discussed in the previous section, we will now describe and discuss four theories about individual behavior change: the Health Belief Model, Self-Efficacy, the Theory of Reasoned Action, and Diffusion of Innovations Theory.[5] We highlight these theories because they contain the models most frequently applied by health promotion practitioners as means to uncover clues that will lead them to the intervention approaches that best fit the problem and circumstances they face. They also fit variously with the predisposing, enabling, and reinforcing factors outlined in Chapter 4 as part of the Precede–Proceed framework for planning. In addition, we present several theories that together seek to explain how change occurs in communities: the Community Coalition Action Theory, Community Capacity, and Social Capital.

In presenting each theory, we will describe a particular health problem ("The Problem"), discuss what the theory says about behavior change in general and about this problem in particular ("The Theory"), and describe the intervention strategies suggested by the theory for addressing this problem ("The Solution").

Health Belief Model

The Problem

Don Weiss is a pediatrician at an urban public health center in St. Louis, Missouri. The center's annual needs assessment showed that immunization rates among children aged two years and younger were very low—fewer than half were fully immunized. Don knew something had to be done, but he wasn't sure what. At the next staff meeting, he asked several staff members to work with him in addressing the problem. He told them, "We've got to know why parents aren't bringing their kids in for shots. If we know the reasons, we can try to do something about it."

For several weeks, Don and his staff made it a point to interview personally all new parents who came into the center for any reason. They also interviewed by telephone a number of the center's patients who had children aged two and younger. They wanted to know what factors influenced parents' decisions to have their children immunized. When Don and his colleagues compared their notes after the next staff meeting, several clear patterns emerged:

- Parents did not know when and how many shots were recommended.
- Parents said their children looked healthy, and therefore must not need shots.
- Parents believed that childhood diseases were just a part of growing up, and not something serious.
- Working parents could not get to the health center during its hours of operation.
- There were few public transportation routes to the health center.
- Compared to other demands and concerns, immunization just wasn't a high priority.

The Theory

The Health Belief Model (HBM) suggests that unless a person sees some value in making a behavior change, there will be no reason for him or her even to consider the change.[6] The HBM emphasizes four variables: perceived susceptibility, perceived severity, perceived barriers, and perceived benefits. In short, this theory suggests that behavior change is most likely to occur when a person believes he or she is at risk for a particular disease or health problem (perceived susceptibility), believes the consequences of getting that disease would be serious for him or her (perceived severity), and believes that the benefits to be gained from changing the behavior (perceived benefits) outweigh the problems to be overcome in changing the behavior (perceived barriers).

For Don Weiss and the problem of childhood immunization, the HBM seemed to be a good fit. Many parents thought their babies didn't need shots (low perceived susceptibility) and viewed getting an immunizable childhood disease (e.g., measles or mumps) as no big deal (low perceived severity). The center's hours weren't convenient for many parents, and public transportation to the clinic was limited (perceived barriers).

The Solution

According to the HBM, any program that Don Weiss and his staff developed to promote childhood immunization should incorporate the following tactics:

- **Increase perceived susceptibility.** Help parents realize that their children may be at risk for preventable childhood diseases, even if they seem healthy.
- **Increase perceived severity.** Help parents understand that childhood diseases can be very serious and sometimes fatal.

- **Remove perceived barriers (or reduce the perception of barriers as insurmountable).** Adopt evening and/or weekend hours to accommodate working parents; work with the public transportation authority to increase service to the health center.

- **Add perceived benefits (or increase the perception of the actual benefits).** Provide an incentive or reward to parents for their efforts in bringing their children to be immunized; help parents recognize how immunizations protect their children.

Note that if Don Weiss and his staff developed an immunization promotion program that addressed only some of these problems, it might be ineffective. For example, a program that increases the center's hours of operation without changing parents' beliefs that immunizations aren't important would have a limited impact. Although, immunizations would be more accessible, their use would remain low if parents didn't think they were important.

Note also that the beliefs associated with the four dimensions of the HBM constitute predisposing factors in the Precede–Proceed model. It is possible sometimes to alter beliefs about environmental barriers and benefits without actually changing the environment, enabling factors, or reinforcing factors. It is also possible to change the beliefs or perceptions of barriers and benefits by directly changing the enabling and reinforcing factors.

Self-Efficacy

The Problem

Janis Whitlock is the director of the student health center at a large Midwestern university. In addition to providing primary-care services for students, the center offers a variety of educational programs, peer counseling, and an orientation for all incoming freshmen. In the past, Janis and her staff had developed innovative programs to prevent alcohol-related injuries and date rape. Now they face a new challenge. For the third year in a row, the rate of sexually transmitted diseases (STDs) among students reporting symptoms at the student health service has increased. Promoting safe sex practices on campus had always been one of Janis's top priorities, but now the center must do a better job.

With the help of two health education faculty members from the School of Health Sciences, Janis developed a survey to assess students' beliefs and practices about sexual activity and their use of the center's programs. Janis told the faculty members, "Either our programs aren't addressing the real problem, they aren't reaching the students, or both. We need to know where to direct our energy." The anonymous survey was mailed to a random sample of 800 undergraduate students, of whom 468 responded. The survey showed the following results among sexually active students:

- 16 percent said they use a condom every time they have sex.
- 26 percent had initiated a discussion about condom use with a sex partner.
- 79 percent, including 92 percent of females, said that they could not easily discuss condom use with a sex partner.
- 66 percent, including 75 percent of females, said that talking about condom use with a sex partner probably would not make condom use any more acceptable.
- 43 percent of females said that it was likely that asking a sex partner to use a condom would make the partner angry.

The Theory

Self-efficacy is really not a theory itself, but rather an important concept in Bandura's social learning theory.[7] According to social learning theory, individuals who believe they are capable of taking some specific action and who believe that taking that action will lead to a desirable outcome are most likely to change. A person's beliefs about his or her ability to make a particular change are called efficacy expectations or self-efficacy. Beliefs about whether making that change will lead to a particular outcome are called outcome expectations. Both beliefs work together to affect a person's actions. For example, if a person believes that she can make a change but sees no value resulting from her efforts, the chances of her taking action are slim. Likewise, if she believes that making the change would be valuable for her but does not feel capable of making the change, it is unlikely to occur. It is important to note that beliefs about self-efficacy are always specific to some action, not a personality trait. For example, a person may have very high self-efficacy beliefs for changing one behavior, but low self-efficacy beliefs for changing another.

The results from the student survey suggest that the concepts of self-efficacy and outcome expectations may help explain the high rate of STDs that Janis's health center has observed. For sexually active persons, consistent condom use is necessary to prevent the spread of STDs. But, as the survey showed, few students used condoms regularly. Why not? The data shown earlier suggest that many students felt that they weren't able to talk to a partner about condom use (low self-efficacy). Furthermore, many believed that talking to a partner about condom use wouldn't make using condoms any more acceptable, and might even anger some partners (negative outcome expectations). Given these survey results, social learning theory would predict that condom use would be low in this population, and therefore STD rates could be high.

The Solution

Four main factors affect self-efficacy: personal experience, observational experience, verbal persuasion, and physiological state. For example, a student may have high self-efficacy for starting a conversation about condom use because she had done it before (personal experience), because she had attended a class where videotapes and role plays showed other people starting such a conversation (observational experience), because she had been reassured by friends that she could do it (verbal persuasion), or because she didn't get nervous and feel sick when she thought about doing it (no physiological arousal).

Thus, social learning theory would suggest that a program designed to enhance low self-efficacy for negotiating condom use with a sex partner might include some of the following intervention strategies:

- **Teach and model specific behavioral and communication skills for negotiating condom use.** Seeing others demonstrate these skills will help students learn and adopt them.

- **Provide opportunities for students to rehearse these behavioral and communication skills.** Practicing, even in simulations, is valuable experience.

- **Make the initial objectives of the program relatively simple for students to achieve.** For example, an objective might be to ask your partner any one question about condoms the next time you are together. Successes, no matter how small, can help build self-efficacy for future actions. Participants also need to rehearse how to handle this one question because failure, no matter how small, can sometimes discourage them from proceeding to the next step.

- **Focus on the positive aspects of an incomplete performance.** Even in an unsuccessful attempt to initiate discussion about condom use, the student should be able to focus on something positive. Finding and emphasizing that something can offset damage to self-efficacy.

- **Provide reinforcement and encouragement.** Hearing that others believe in you, or think you can do it, builds self-efficacy.

- **Teach relaxation skills.** Students who feel very nervous, become short of breath, or perspire when thinking about talking to a partner about condom use may interpret these signs as meaning they won't be able to do it. Knowing how to calm yourself down can help prevent losing self-efficacy.

To help change negative outcome expectations, a program should clearly demonstrate the relationship between the behavior of interest and the outcome. Where possible, it should provide opportunities for students to experience specific outcomes that may result from the actions they have (or have not) taken. In designing such exercises, it may be especially important to think about the outcomes of a behavior as immediate and tangible, not as long-term health risks or benefits.

In summary, Self-Efficacy fits within the predisposing factors of the Precede–Proceed model, but it can be related to other aspects of social learning theory that fit more clearly under enabling and reinforcing factors.

Theory of Reasoned Action

The Problem

Lincoln Phillips is a graduate student getting a master's degree in public health. For his thesis project, he is working with Forever Yours Senior Center, a large organization that offers programs to more than 2000 senior residents in the Lakewood area adjacent to the university. Lincoln's primary interest is to develop and implement physical activity programs for older adults. Lincoln had seen his grandmother suffer the consequences of osteoporosis, had read about the low rates of physical activity in aging populations, and thought this issue was an area of real need where he could make a difference. As he'd learned in his classes, his first step was to conduct a needs assessment. He spent weeks talking with staff members from agencies and organizations that served older adults, with family members of older adults, and with older adults themselves at the Forever Yours center, in coffee shops, and in their homes. As he completed more and more interviews, Lincoln could see several clear patterns emerging:

- Most older adults believed that, at their age, there was little benefit from physical activity.

- Many older adults reported that their friends and neighbors were not physically active.

- Many older adults and some family members thought of physical activity as jogging or bicycling, as they saw the "young people" in the park doing.

- Many family members of older adults thought physical activity would be dangerous for their relatives.

The Theory

According to the Theory of Reasoned Action, the best predictor of a person taking some health-related action is whether the person intends to take action.[8] The theory specifies that a person's intention is determined by two factors: the person's attitude toward the behavior and what the person thinks other people would want him or her to do regarding the behavior. A person's attitudes are made up of two types of beliefs:

- Beliefs about outcomes that may result from engaging in the behavior

- Beliefs about how desirable or undesirable those outcomes are

A person's perceptions of others' beliefs are determined by two factors:

- What the person thinks others would like him or her to do regarding the behavior
- How much or little the person wants to comply with what others think he or she should do

In summary, when a person believes that a behavior will lead to some valuable outcome and that others whom that person respects and wants to please think he or she should engage in the behavior, then the person is more likely to intend to take action and, therefore, is more likely to act.

Lincoln remembered the Theory of Reasoned Action from his classes on behavior change theory and saw that it really applied to his project with the senior center. Many of the older adults with whom he spoke saw little benefit to be gained from doing physical activity, and some even thought it could hurt them. Clearly, they had a negative attitude toward physical activity. In addition, few of their friends and neighbors were physically active, and some members of their families thought exercising could be risky for them. If the older adults valued or respected the opinions of their friends and family members, this factor would also undermine any attempt he made to promote physical activity with this population.

The Solution

Lincoln realized that, among other things, the program he developed would need to address older adults' negative attitudes toward physical activity and their perceptions of how the important people in their lives felt about them doing physical activity. Reviewing the Theory of Reasoned Action, he saw several possible solutions. To change older adults' attitudes about physical activity, he could:

- **Add a new, positive belief.** "Physical activity like walking is safe and beneficial, can be a social activity with friends, and can reduce your risk of injury by making your body stronger."
- **Reinforce an existing positive belief.** "Remember how much you used to enjoy a more active lifestyle? Regular physical activity can help you become that way again."
- **Challenge an existing negative belief.** "You think you're too old to exercise, but doctors and other health experts say it's one of the best things you can do for yourself, no matter what your age."
- **Enhance the perceived desirability of a new or existing belief.** "The stronger you are, the less you'll have to rely on others, the longer you'll be able to live independently, and the more you can play with your grandchildren."

To change older adults' beliefs about what others want them to do, he could:

- **Change the attitudes of the important others.** Help family members and friends recognize the value of physical activity for older adults, and ask them to support and encourage their efforts to be more active.

- **Add new "others" to their lives.** Introduce new social contacts, such as members of a mall walking club, a doctor, or a pharmacist, who support physical activity.

- **Challenge their beliefs about what others think they should do.** "Actually, your friends, your family, and your doctor all think it would be a good idea for you to become more active—why don't you ask them?"

- **Change the motivation to comply with others.** "You shouldn't be so concerned about what Mr. Jones thinks; your doctor and your family think it's a good idea for you to be physically active."

Diffusion of Innovations Theory

The Problem

One month later, Lincoln had developed a comprehensive physical activity program for the Forever Yours Senior Center based on the combination of (1) the insight he gained about the attitudes of seniors by using the Theory of Reasoned Action and (2) intervention ideas he received as a result of correspondence with Drs. Michael Pratt and Carl Casperson, physical activity experts at the CDCP. Lincoln shared his proposed program with his faculty advisor, who concurred that his use of the Theory of Reasoned Action was indeed appropriate. The advisor then added, "Is there anything else you might do to maximize the chance that the seniors will actually undertake the activities you are now prepared to offer?"

As Lincoln prepared his response, the professor said, "Take another look at the Diffusion of Innovations Theory and see if any ideas crop up."

The Theory

The Diffusion of Innovations Theory has its origins in communications and, interestingly, agriculture.[9] It explains how, over time, a new idea or product (an innovation) gains momentum and spreads (diffuses) through a given population. *Adoption* is a key word in the context of this theory—simply translated, it means to do something (e.g., think, believe, purchase, act, or behave) in a way that you haven't previously. Thus, new ideas and products spread in a population or society to the extent that people "adopt" them. The notion of an adoption spreading through a population implies, of course, that not everyone jumps on the bandwagon immediately. Some do; others, however, are more conservative and wait it out, perhaps looking for evidence that the innovation in question is not just a passing fancy.

Researchers have noted that those who adopt an innovation early in the diffusion process seem to demonstrate characteristics that are different from those who adopt with the majority, and they differ still more from those who adopt even later. Individuals who are the first to take up a new idea, product, or action are called innovators; they are followed, in order, by early adopters, the early majority, the later majority, and finally the late adopters (sometimes unkindly labeled laggards). Generally, simple exposure to and a reasonable level of comprehension of the innovation is sufficient to trigger adoption by innovators. The level of effort required to predict adoption becomes incrementally greater for those in the early-adopter, early-majority, and later-majority groups.

Examples of adopting an innovation within the commercial sector include purchasing a color TV in 1970, a CD player in 1980, and a cellular phone in 1990. Examples in the health sector would include seeking out influenza vaccinations in 1970, purchasing and drinking skim milk in 1980, and passing indoor clean air policies and tobacco excise tax legislation in 1990.

As you will note in the examples given, some adoption decisions have effects beyond the individual level. As Glanz and Rimer so correctly point out, when teachers adopt a new school health curriculum, when a work-site manager contracts for new screening services, and when a city council adopts a recycling policy, the implications obviously extend far beyond the individual.[10]

An important aspect of this theory for practitioners is that five characteristics about the innovation itself appear to have a strong influence on the extent to which the product or recommended action will be adopted. Table 5.1 provides a definition of each of these characteristics and an explanation of how, if left unattended, each characteristic could inhibit adoption.

Practitioners who understand the theory of adoption routinely test their program ideas against these characteristics—after all, a brilliant, scientifically and theoretically sound idea won't be used if the intended users see it as too complicated and potentially at odds with their values. For example, the Washington Heights–Inwood Heart Health Program is a community-based heart disease prevention program serving a low-income community population of 240,000 people in inner-city New York. In reporting their six-year evaluation results, researchers described a comprehensive "low-fat milk campaign" (involving school, community, and policy components) that was remarkably successful in lowering the intake of saturated fat among children in the community. In describing the factors contributing to the success of the intervention, the investigators said:

> The recommended behavioral change was easy to understand and simple to do, did not impose time commitments or significant monetary costs, was readily accepted by children, involved fun and interactive campaign activities, and emphasized positive messages and social reinforcements in campaign themes (p. 167).[11]

TABLE 5.1   Diffusion of Innovations Theory

Concept	Definition	Reasons for Not Adopting
Relative advantage	The degree to which an innovation is seen as better than the idea, practice, program, or product it replaces	Benefits not evident (e.g., no apparent savings, doesn't give me more than I have, doesn't save time)
Compatibility	How consistent the innovation is with values, habits, experience, and needs of potential adopters	Not consistent with my values (e.g., I believe in the right to bear arms and your policy restricts my ability to buy guns)
Complexity	How difficult the innovation is to understand and/or use	Too complicated (e.g., I can't do your weight-loss program because it means I have to get a babysitter)
Trialability	The extent to which the innovation can be experimented with before a commitment to adopt is required	You won't let me see if I like it, so no thanks; will you guarantee it?
Observability	The extent to which the innovation provides tangible or visible results	How do I know it will work; I don't see anyone else doing it

The Solution

Lincoln asked for and received permission from the Forever Yours Senior Center director to make arrangements to meet with several groups of senior participants. He scheduled three small-group sessions including about 10 seniors per group. In leisurely settings that included coffee, tea, and cookies, Lincoln carried on a discussion with each group that lasted an hour or so. After appropriate introductions, he described the activities that were likely to be included in the program and then structured the discussions so that he could get a sense of the seniors' reactions based on the five concepts described in Table 5.1.

Relative Advantage.   He discovered that some of the seniors wondered whether the effort was really "worth it." As Lincoln briefly described some of the benefits of physical activity to the seniors, he noted that a large number were unaware of the fact that exercising had direct benefits for them "even at this late stage." As a result, he thought of several possible tactics:

1. Have a doctor and/or physical therapist visit with the seniors and their families to discuss the numerous benefits of exercise to this age group. For example, many conditions can be prevented or their symptoms reduced by engaging in appropriate exercise (thereby resulting in fewer visits to the doctor and less frequent hospitalization), and physiological changes resulting from exercise can increase feelings of physical and mental well-being (thereby improving mood and relieving symptoms of depression). The speaker could reassure the audience about the safety of exercise and suggest that those who have specific health concerns have a simple and routine medical check with their doctor before the programs commence.

2. Have a social worker or member of the clergy talk to the seniors about the benefits of the social aspects of exercise, including friendship, team building, and the enrichment of community life.

3. Assistance from the "opinion leaders" in the Forever Yours Senior Center can be enlisted to maximize members' attendance at these presentations, and later to generate discussion and active participation in aspects of program implementation. This goal can be achieved through informal channels using established social networks within the center. The higher the level of members' early involvement in priority setting and suggesting how the programs might best be run, the higher the participation rates will be.

Compatibility.   Lincoln found that seniors wanted the activity program to "fit in" with their lifestyles, interests, and abilities. Some of the activities could encompass or expand upon things that the seniors were already doing in their daily lives (e.g., walking to shops instead of taking the bus).

He also found out that the social aspects of a proposed program were very important. Therefore, it would be useful to incorporate an opportunity for socializing, perhaps over tea or coffee, after some of the activities. In fact, some people implied that such social contact was more attractive to them than the physical activity. This insight triggered the following ideas:

1. Offer a variety of programs, as people differ widely in the types of exercise that appeal to them. Activities such as dancing and cycling, for example, might have particular appeal to many seniors because they may well have had good experiences with them in their younger days or view them as truly recreational. Other factors necessitating a variety of programs are the weather, as certain activities may be impractical or lack appeal on cool or wet days, and the fact that some activities may be unsuitable for people with particular medical conditions. Options might include the following:

   • Graded walks in groups, where the exercise is combined with social interaction

- Ballroom or "old-time" dancing evenings
- Exercise classes such as "Fun and Fitness for the Over-60s," including riding (stationary) exercise bicycles and a variety of other exercises
- Swimming

2. Regularly consult members to determine which types of activity are of interest, and ask the "opinion leaders" to encourage suggestions and discussion on the issues involved.

Complexity.   Most participants did not find Lincoln's proposed activities to be too complex. However, they did express concern about their friends whose mobility was seriously impaired and who were restricted to wheelchairs or walkers. What could be done to make activities amenable to them as well? As he thought about this concern, no good ideas came to Lincoln's mind. In truth, he knew little about physical activities for handicapped senior citizens. He made a mental note to consult with his professor and with a friend who was a physical therapy student.

Trialability.   In each of the three discussion groups, at least one or two people had expressed a desire to "test the waters" with the activities, without pressure or obligation and before any commitment to sign up was required. Several thoughts came to Lincoln's mind:

- Offer participation in the activity for an initial trial period, making it clear that there is no obligation to continue taking part afterward.
- Provide an incentive to come to the first session (e.g., discounts at the local sports clothing retailer, grocery store, or pharmacy).
- Provide home pickups and return transportation.

Observability.   During the discussions, participants raised three questions:

1. Were they the first ones to try this kind of activity?
2. Were there really visible benefits from the innovations Lincoln was proposing?
3. Were they more likely to participate in them?

Lincoln thought of several ways he might address these questions:

- Enlist the help of members of the Forever Yours Senior Center or members of the public who have reaped the benefits of exercise, and who are willing to give short talks to members about how it has changed their lives in measurable ways (e.g., weight loss, reduced blood pressure, increased stamina, more mobility resulting in fewer arthritic symptoms). Appropriate photographs or slides of "before and after" may be useful in illustrating these messages.

- Later, when programs have been running for some time, recruit "innovators" and "early adopters" to give these talks, and to discuss and demonstrate their successes in less formal settings within the center's social networks, so as to increase program participation rates.

- When promoting or advertising the programs, display photographs on bulletin boards of groups of seniors taking part in the activities (from other centers, towns, or states) to demonstrate that other seniors' groups already run these programs and find them enjoyable. For example, photographs of happy groups at a social dance or groups of seniors walking and talking in a shady park could appeal to many people and induce them to join up.

- To be able to quantify the benefits of exercise, it is useful to encourage participants to keep a simple record of some measurements over time (e.g., weight, distance walked with ease, time taken to swim a certain distance). These records help to demonstrate objectively the improvements gained by program participation and can be used to encourage others to take part.

COMMUNITY CAPACITY, COALITION-BUILDING, AND SOCIAL CAPITAL THEORIES

The Problem

Town A and Town B are very similar. Both are Midwestern towns with similar demographics and a population of about 20,000. The two are geographically near one another, so the climate, industrial base, and rural/urban split are almost identical in the two communities.

Scratching the surface, though, you would notice some interesting differences between Town A and Town B. Town A has many residents who have lived there all their lives—and are the third or fourth generation to do so. People who went away to school tend to come back, after finding that they missed the small-town atmosphere. If you ask people why, they are likely to cite a number of different reasons, but it all boils down to this: In Town A, people cooperate and give each other the benefit of the doubt. The community has its share of problems, like any other modern place. Even so, people seem to be able to set aside their differences and work together to tackle these problems. The town's schools, places of worship, private and public health institutions, and elected officials have a track record of working together—a track record that allows them to compete successfully on the national stage.

In Town B, a similar profile has yielded very different sentiments. If you ask people about the town's problems, they sound resigned. "It's always been this way," they might say. People have long memories about what has gone wrong in the past: a corrupt former mayor, his cronies at the newspaper and police department, community groups in fierce competition with one another. Levels of trust are low, and optimism is even more scarce.

Many places have pockets with the characteristics of each of these situations: some individuals and organizations who work together well and thrive, and others that are characterized by mistrust and destructive competition. Sometimes, as in Towns A and B, one set of circumstances will take hold—for better or worse—and will shape how people perceive their community as a whole, its potential, and their place in it.

What does this state have to do with community health promotion? Everything. If we see the community as both a context for health improvement and an essential ingredient of making health improvement possible, we need to know everything we can about a community's capacity and social capital, and how these factors may affect the work and progress of coalitions within a community. Several emerging theories offer tantalizing insights about these key ingredients and, best of all, suggest that there are effective ways of improving a community's prospects. Town B, in other words, can become more like Town A.

The Theories

Community Coalition Action Theory

Coalitions are a common feature of community health improvement efforts. Sometimes they arise naturally—for example, when many different organizations share an interest in one topic, such as children's health. In other situations, they are mandated by funders who believe that multiple perspectives yield benefits such as representation and sustainability.

Over the past several decades, many communities have documented their experiences working with coalitions or other collaborative efforts. Until recently, however, the benefits of coalitions and the factors leading to their success (or, in many cases, their failure) did not receive much scrutiny.

The Community Coalition Action Theory[12] fills this gap by analyzing the processes and outcomes that are unique to coalitions. The theory's key insight is that coalitions move through different stages, not unlike the Stages of Change that characterize individual behavior change. In the model, these are described as formation, maintenance, and institutionalization.

In the *formation* stage, a coalition is created by a convener or lead agency that recruits an initial group of members. Together, these members then create structures and procedures to carry out the coalition's work.

In the *maintenance* stage, the coalition undertakes the hard work of assessing, planning, selecting, and implementing strategies—all the while meeting the considerable challenge of keeping its members engaged and active. This phase is often a danger zone for coalitions. If the planning and implementation tasks are not effective, members may lose interest and commitment, making it even more difficult to recover and move forward. On the other hand, coalitions that overcome the natural hurdles posed by the maintenance stage can look forward to a track record of success that, for many, becomes a self-fulfilling prophecy.

In the *institutionalization* stage, a coalition has addressed its initial work so successfully that it either becomes an institution itself or its work is adopted by others in the community.

Community Capacity

A community's capacity to change for the better is relevant to many fields, but has particular appeal for those interested in improving health status. What makes a community tick? How can its strengths or assets be tapped, and its deficiencies addressed? What are the dimensions of community capacity?

A recent review of community capacity research[13] identified several of these dimensions:

- Skills, knowledge, and resources—such as strategic planning and group process skills or other assets

- The nature of social relationships—the networks and ties within a community

- Structures and mechanisms for community dialogue—voluntary associations, collaborative groups and coalitions, and other "convener" or catalytic organizations such as community foundations or task forces

- Leadership—a combination of communication, analysis and judgment, coaching, visioning, trust building, teamwork, reflection and learning, and partnerships

- Civic participation—citizen involvement, representation, voice, power sharing and structures

- Value systems—a community's norms, standards, and expectations regarding core values such as equity, participation, collaboration, inclusion, and collective responsibility

- Learning culture—self-awareness, institutional memory, and an ability to learn from the past (instead of wallowing in it or blaming each other)

Community capacity alone cannot lead to change, but it may be an essential ingredient that dictates how quickly change occurs and how long it lasts. It is also important to note that community capacity is both an input and an output of community efforts. The more a community struggles and succeeds, the more capacity it will have for future efforts. For all these reasons, a community's current and potential capacity are essential pieces of information for those planning community health interventions.[14]

Social Capital

Social capital refers to the process of people and organizations within a community working collaboratively, in an atmosphere of trust, toward the accomplishment of mutual social benefit. Efforts to measure social capital have been part of many fields, including the sociological, educational, and political science literature. One of the most frequently referenced scholars studying social capital is Robert Putnam, a professor of political science at Harvard.[15] He has defined social capital as the processes among people that establish networks, norms, and social trust, and facilitate coordination and cooperation for mutual benefit.

The foundation for Putnam's ideas about social capital was influenced in part by his study of local governments in Italy from 1970 to 1990.[16] In 1970, a new set of regional governments was established in Italy, all of which—on paper at least—had comparable organizational structures and adequate resources in relative terms. Putnam's research revealed that two decades after the 1970 reorganization, some rather dramatic differences existed among some of the communities. One group of communities was very inefficient—they were corrupt, tended to be managed on the basis of favors to small special-interest groups, and appeared to invest little in civic improvement and development programs. Others operated under more democratic and interdependent principles, and civic programs such as arts and sports groups, day-care centers, industrial parks, job programs, and family clinics were much more visible.

Putnam concluded that the more efficient and effective governments were those where citizens demonstrated high levels of what he termed "civic engagement." Indicators of civic engagement were manifested by rather common acts of social investment: voter turnout, newspaper readership, and participation in cooperative groups such as sporting clubs, parent/teacher organizations, local arts and theater activities, and so on. Putnam observed that central to these civic actions was a sense of social trust.

The critical elements of social capital include the following:

- Trust
- Cooperation/coordination
- Civic engagement
- Reciprocity

These elements overlap with aspects of both coalition-building and community capacity. In particular, the elements of trust, cooperation/coordination, and reciprocity are features of the social and organizational interactions that make coalitions succeed. Likewise, these elements and civic engagement are prominent in dimensions of community capacity.

More recently, researchers have explored two levels of social capital that tie it even more strongly to coalition-building and overall community capacity.[17] The first is bonding social capital, defined as the sociocultural milieu that nurtures the group solidarity typical in Town A. The other is bridging social capital, which can be thought of as similar to institutional infrastructure. Bridging social capital can be detected at the organizational level where norms, values, and social structures facilitate broader connections. Clearly, though, bridging and bonding social capital overlap, in that individuals participate in social networks both on their own and as representatives of organizations.

The Solutions

Suppose Town B is seeking a large grant to address a community health problem, but the grant asks for information on the community's coalition-building experience, overall capacity, and social capital. What can Town B do to compete for this grant and to set the stage for becoming more like Town A? How can the theories described previously guide its actions?

First, people in Town B who are interested in change can try to conduct a candid assessment of their community in terms of coalition-building potential, overall community capacity, and both bridging and bonding social capital. Regardless of the measures and forums they choose for this assessment, they should work hard to avoid the blame-casting that has marred previous discussions ("Back in 1972, the mayor said this, so we'll never trust any mayor ever again . . ."). While candor is a goal, so is achieving enough of a clean slate to move forward. These two elements—constructive assessments and looking ahead instead of dwelling on the past—could eventually take root as new community norms.

In seeking the grant, the members of Town B's emerging coalition should point out that after this candid assessment, they realize that they need help at a different stage than do other communities. (In other words, they should appeal to the funder to invest in moving Town B along a continuum toward more capacity and social capital.) For example, there is no shame in admitting that their coalition may be at an earlier formation stage than others, requiring different talents and resources. Town B residents might even consider the parallels between their situation as a community and that of an individual moving through the Stages of Change.[18] For example:

Precontemplation. With some exceptions, many residents of Town B could be described as precontemplatives. They believe that Town B has always had strife and conflict, and probably always will. Previous attempts to change the town's economic profile have either failed or led to discord among residents.

Contemplation. A first step out of precontemplation would involve an open discussion of problems, perhaps led by local news organizations, that sought to define reality in a balanced way, avoiding the blame and recrimination that seem to characterize many accounts of past events in Town B. It would be very important to highlight the town's many assets in such a discussion and not dwell on the negative legacy. In short, the leadership task would be to define and address Town B's realities.

Preparation.   To prepare for future action and sustained change, key groups within the town should be identified to help find middle ground and move toward greater inclusiveness. Community forums could be convened in which information from the previous stage is discussed and used to create a positive, meaningful vision of Town B's future. Specific tasks might include learning how to agree to disagree in communitywide forums and keeping one another mindful of avoiding personal attacks and blame for things that go wrong. The goal of this stage would be to agree to try new collaborative efforts, realizing that they may be difficult and painful at first.

Action.   Collaborative efforts, however flawed or hesitant, would be launched. The goals would be to create stronger norms for valuing collaboration. Individuals and organizations would specifically be asked (and be willing) to give up turf and act in good faith regarding others' motives. As a result, social capital markers such as volunteerism, levels of trust, and civic engagement would increase over time.

Maintenance.   Town B's residents would now acknowledge the benefits of a more collaborative, trusting approach. Over time, peer pressure to maintain collaborative approaches and coalitions would emerge as a reinforcement of collaborative behavior (and as a disincentive for those who relapse into negative behavior). As collaboration becomes the norm, more examples of success will emerge, making more individuals and organizations willing to take the risk of collaborating with others for the collective good of the town.

Communities, like people, can move through stages that may sometimes feel much like "one step forward, two steps back." With awareness and persistence, however, both individuals and communities can acquire the skills and insights that allow them to move forward, building the capacity to try and then sustain change. The theories described here show how an understanding of theoretical models can guide us as we choose interventions as well as the structures and processes that support them.

SUMMARY

We have all heard Kurt Lewin's oft-cited aphorism that there is nothing so practical as a good theory. This leads us to make at least two assumptions: (1) "good theories" exist, and (2) those theories are sufficiently well understood to be put to use.

In practical terms, theories are "good" to the extent that they help us understand how things work. Ample empirical research indicates that theories give us clues, some of which are highly predictive, of the key factors, forces, and conditions that influence health status and health behaviors. Our counsel to practitioners is to become familiar with those theories and their elements and to continually use that knowledge to probe for the little insights could make big differences in the effects of a health promotion program. Xiao Fang was using such a probe when her new understanding of Stages of Change theory prompted her to wonder: "If a large number of men in the Eastern District are not in the ready for action stage, an extensive campaign on smoking cessation may not be a good investment of time and effort." For Xiao Fang, a good theory was indeed practical.

As more research in community health promotion is undertaken, more theories will come to light. As long as health promotion practitioners view theories as useful and practical tools, they will be readily incorporated into more robust and effective programs. In the next chapter on tactics, notice how the application of theory influences decisions regarding intervention strategies and tactics.

ENDNOTES

1. By using the Stages of Change example, we are not saying that it is the best or even the most appropriate theory to use in Li Fang's case. We use this example to illustrate how a working knowledge of theory can influence decisions made when one is planning an outcome-oriented health promotion program. As our awareness of various theories expands, so too does our professional responsibility to justify our preference for one theory over another or to combine the most relevant elements of several theories. For added information on Stages of Change theories, we suggest the writing of James Prochaska, beginning with: Prochaska JO, DiClemente CC, Norcross JC. In search of how people change: applications to addictive behaviors. *Am Psychologist.* 1992;47:1102–1114. A recent exploration of change theories can also be found in Weinstein ND, Sandman PM. The precaution adoption process model and its application. In: DiClemente RJ, Crosby RA, Kegler MC, eds. *Emerging Theories in Health Promotion Practice and Research: Strategies for Improving Public Health.* San Francisco: Jossey-Bass; 2002.

2. World No-Tobacco Day is an annual event that encourages governments, communities, and other groups to become aware of the hazards of tobacco and encourages those who use tobacco to quit for at least one day. Children's Day is a Chinese holiday celebrating the importance of nurturing children.

3. Glanz K, Rimer BK. *Theory at a Glance: A Guide for Health Promotion Practice.* Washington, DC: U.S. Department of Health and Human Services, National Institutes of Health; 1986:11.

4. For basic readings in the fundamental principles of community organization and participation, we recommend Alinsky SD. *Reveille for Radicals.* Chicago: University of Chicago; 1969; and Freire P. *Education for Critical Consciousness.* New York: Sebury Press; 1973. For direct health promotion applications of those principles, we suggest Minkler M. Improving health through community organization. In: Glanz K, Marcus-Lewis F, Rimer B, eds. *Health Behavior and Education: Theory, Research and Practice.* San Francisco: Jossey-Bass; 1990.

5. The Transtheoretical Model, or Stages of Change theory, is a frequently applied thesis in health promotion. It is not included here because it is a component in the "Old Horse" case story.

6. For background reading on the Health Belief Model, we suggest Becker MH, ed. The health belief model and personal health behavior. *Health Education Monographs.* 1974;2:324–473; Rosenstock IM. Historical origins of the health belief model. *Health Education Monographs.* 1974;2:470–473; Janz NK, Becker MH. The health belief model: a decade later. *Health Educ Q.* 1984;11:1–47; and Becker MH, Haefner D, Kasl SV, et al. Selected psychosocial models and correlates of individual health-related behaviors. *Med Care.* 1977; 15(suppl):27–46. See also Fisher J, Fisher W. The information-motivation-behavioral skills model. In: DiClemente RJ, Crosby RA, Kegler MC, eds. *Emerging Theories in Health Promotion Practice and Research: Strategies for Improving Public Health.* San Francisco: Jossey-Bass; 2002.

7. For background reading on social learning theory, we suggest Bandura A. Toward a unifying theory of behavior change. *Psychological Review.* 1977;84(2): 191–215; Bandura A. *Social Foundations of Thought and Action.* Englewood Cliffs, NJ: Prentice-Hall; 1986; and Strecker VJ, DeVillis BM, Becker MH, Rosenstock IM. The role of self efficacy in achieving health behavior change. *Health Educ Q.* 1986;13:73–92.

8. For further reading on the Theory of Reasoned Action, we suggest Ajzen I, Fishbein M. *Understanding Attitudes and Predicting Social Behavior.* Englewood Cliffs, NJ: Prentice-Hall; 1980; and Jorgenson SR, Sonstegard JS. Predicting adolescent sexual and contraceptive behavior: an application and test to the Fishbein model. *J Marriage Family.* 1984;46:43–55. See also Fisher J, Fisher W. The information-motivation-behavioral skills model. In: DiClemente RJ, Crosby RA, Kegler MC, eds. *Emerging Theories in Health Promotion Practice and Research: Strategies for Improving Public Health.* San Francisco: Jossey-Bass; 2002.

9. For further reading on the Diffusion of Innovations Theory, we suggest Rogers EM. *The Diffusion of Innovations,* 3rd ed. New York: Free Press; 1983; Basch CD, Eveland JD, Portnoy B. Diffusion systems for education and learning about health. *Family and Community Health.* 1986;9:1–26; and Orlandi MA. The diffusion and adoption of worksite health promotion innovations: an analysis of barriers. *Preventive Medicine.* 1987;16:119–130.

10. Glanz K, Rimer BK. *Theory at a Glance: A Guide for Health Promotion Practice.* Washington, DC: U.S. Department of Health and Human Services, National Institutes of Health; 1986.

11. Shea S, Basch C, Wechsler H, Lantiqua R. The Washington Heights–Inwood healthy heart program: a 6-year report from a disadvantaged urban setting. *AJPH.* 1996;86(2):166–171.

12. Butterfoss FD, Kegler MC. Toward a comprehensive understanding of community coalitions: moving from practice to theory. In: DiClemente RJ, Crosby RA, Kegler MC, eds. *Emerging Theories in Health Promotion Practice and Research: Strategies for Improving Public Health.* San Francisco: Jossey-Bass; 2002.

13. Norton BL, McLeroy KR, Burdine JN, Felix MRJ, Doresey AM. Community capacity: concept, theory, and methods. In: DiClemente RJ, Crosby RA, Kegler MC, eds. *Emerging Theories in Health Promotion Practice and Research: Strategies for Improving Public Health.* San Francisco: Jossey-Bass; 2002.

14. For more information on measuring community capacity and social capital, see:

> Eng E, Parker E. Measuring community competence in the Mississippi Delta: the interface between program evaluation and empowerment. *Health Educ Q.* 1994;21(2):199–220.
>
> Buckner J. The development of an instrument to measure neighborhood cohesion. *J Comm Psychology.* 1988;16(6):771–790.
>
> Wickizer T, VonKorff M, Cheadle A, et al. Activating communities for health promotion: a process of evaluation method. *Am J Public Health.* 1993;83:561–567.
>
> Fawcett S, Francisco W, Paine-Andrews A, et al. *Work Group Evaluation Handbook: Evaluating and Supporting Community Interventions for Health and Development.* Published by the Work Group for Health and Community Development, 1486 Dole Center, Kansas University, Lawrence, KS 66045.
>
> Social Capital Assessment Tool (SCAT). Available from www.worldbank.org/poverty/scapital/index.htm.
>
> Social Capital Community Benchmark Survey. Available from www.cfsv.org/communitysurvey.
>
> Stone W. *Measuring Social Capital: Towards a Theoretically Informed Measurement Framework of Researching Social Capital in Family and Community Life* (www.aifs.org.au/institute/pubs/stone.html).

15. Putnam R. The prosperous community: social capital and public life. *American Prospect.* 1993;143:35–42.

16. Putnam R. *Making Democracy Work: Civic Traditions in Modern Italy.* Princeton, NJ: Princeton University Press; 1993.

17. For a more extensive discussion of bridging and bonding social capital, see Kreuter MW, Lezin N. Social capital theory: implications for community-based health promotion. In: DiClemente RJ, Crosby RA, Kegler MC, eds. *Emerging Theories in Health Promotion Practice and Research: Strategies for Improving Public Health.* San Francisco: Jossey-Bass; 2002.

18. Adapted from Kreuter MW, Lezin N. Social capital theory: implications for community-based health promotion. In: DiClemente RJ, Crosby RA, Kegler MC, eds. *Emerging Theories in Health Promotion Practice and Research: Strategies for Improving Public Health.* San Francisco: Jossey-Bass; 2002.

CHAPTER 6

Tactics

Case Story
CHECKMATE

Everyone in the family looked forward to the annual Thanksgiving gathering at the Rodriguez home in Salinas, California. Edgar and Carla Rodriguez had three children: two daughters, one son, and a 10-month-old grandchild, Esther. This year's gathering was special because Ray, Edgar and Carla's son, was coming home from Germany for the first time in two years.

Outside the Rodriguez household, Ray was known as Captain Raymond E. Rodriguez, U.S. Air Force. He had gone to Fresno State University on a football scholarship but suffered a career-ending knee injury in his sophomore year. It was during his rehabilitation that he discovered his interest in the field of physical therapy. After graduating and completing his training as a certified physical therapist, he accepted a commission in the Air Force. Ray specialized in rehabilitating patients suffering from mission- and work-related injuries; in the process, he distinguished himself not only as a superb practitioner, but also as a first-rate administrator. Ray was a "people person" who had the ability to combine science and humanity without losing perspective on either one. Nearly 10 years of working on the restorative side of health in the Air Force had firmed up Ray's desire to become more involved in prevention.

Two months before Thanksgiving, Ray received news that he had been selected to provide leadership for and direct an Air Force Health and Wellness Center (HAWC). Air Force policy calls for one of these centers to be established at every Air Force installation for the purpose of providing planned programs in health promotion and disease prevention for active-duty personnel, military retirees, their dependents, and civilian employees. It was the right job at the right time for Ray; his assignment was taking him from Wiesbaden, Germany, to Dobbins Air Force Base just outside Atlanta, Georgia.

During the Thanksgiving holiday, Ray rediscovered the reality of family life: tight sleeping quarters, chairs squeezed around the dinner table, lines for the bathroom, a few debates about who was going to be responsible for what, too much food, and a house full of people who couldn't care less about their wild-looking morning hair! He marveled at how five days of such joyful chaos relieved the tension in his body.

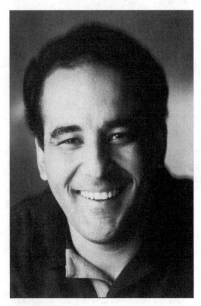

Ray Rodriguez

As always, the good-byes were tearful. Ray anticipated the stress that would be caused by hordes of travelers. After negotiating the holiday traffic on the two-hour drive from Salinas to San Francisco International Airport and enduring the usual scheduling delays, he finally settled into his seat for his flight to Atlanta.

*   *   *

Colonel Tim Gayle, chief of health promotion activities and programs for the entire U.S. Air Force, had sent Ray a packet of materials to review in preparation for a two-day seminar on health promotion for all HAWC directors in the southeastern region. Just after takeoff, Ray reached down for his briefcase under the seat in front of him, extracted a stack of articles, picked one out, and started to read, making occasional notes in the margins.

Although Ray was gregarious and made friends easily, he had learned that most travelers like the privacy of their space, so he had made it a habit not to initiate conversation on an airplane. But after a few minutes, the woman sitting next to him asked, "Excuse me, are you involved with health reform?"

Ray shrugged his shoulders, "Oh, well, not directly—why do you ask?"

"I couldn't help seeing the title of that article, 'Planning for Health Promotion,' and I just thought . . ."

Ray politely interrupted with a chuckle, "Well, I am in the health field." He went on to explain that he was catching up on some reading for a briefing he was going to have about his new assignment at Dobbins Air Force Base. He stuck out his hand. "I'm Ray Rodriguez."

"Lela Davis. Nice to meet you, Ray."

"Are you in the health field as well?" Ray asked.

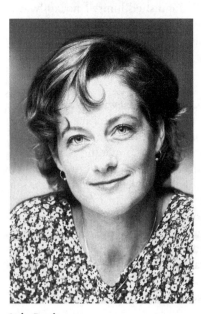

Lela Davis

"No, I've been involved with city planning for over 10 years, the last five of which have been in Atlanta; actually, I'm a demographer by training!" Lela gestured to the flight attendant.

"May I have a cup of coffee, please?"

"Cream and sugar?"

"Just cream, thank you," Lela said.

The flight attendant looked at Ray. "And you, sir?"

Ray held up the palm of his hand. "I'm fine, thanks." Ray enjoyed the art of conversation. At that very moment, he would rather exchange thoughts with Lela than plow through his readings! In just a few minutes, it became clear that Ray and Lela shared a common interest in strategic planning.

During the course of their casual conversation, Lela commented, "During the time I've worked on community planning, the most interesting and practical interpretation of strategic planning was given to me by a friend who is an accomplished chess player."

"Not that guy who beat the computer?" Ray asked.

"Kasparov?" Lela chuckled. "No, not him. Do you play chess?"

"Used to," Ray said pensively, "but I haven't played in years." He thought of his early teen years in Salinas, when his father had taught him to play with a set of chess pieces carved out of shiny marble. But along with many other small pleasures, chess had given way to football.

Lela went on, "Anyway, here's what my chess player friend said: When accomplished players start the game, neither player is certain of the approach his or her opponent is going to take. So, in the beginning, the players are basically checking each other out—looking for possible openings and clues on what to do next. Their interpretation of these clues leads to the formulation of their overall plan or strategy. When they are confident of their strategic plan, it is simply a matter of applying the specific tactics most likely to lead to the capture of the queen."

Ray grinned and nodded. "So, in other words, strategic planning is what you do when you don't know what to do; tactics are what you do when you know what to do!"

Lela laughed. "Right on, Captain! But, as is usually the case, the devil is in the details."

"Meaning?" Ray asked.

Lela took a sip of her coffee. "Meaning that when you're dealing with the kind of planning that both of us do—involving people with differing beliefs, politics, and views—cookie-cutter approaches won't get the job done. You have to be flexible and strategic with your tactics. In the kind of community planning I do, I have found that even the most tried-and-true methods have to be adapted to the unique needs of a community or neighborhood." That made sense to Ray.

The flight to Atlanta was a smooth one. Ray reflected on his conversation with Lela—how perfectly the chess metaphor explained the process he followed as a physical therapist. First, a team of health workers diagnosed and assessed the extent of injury and trauma suffered by a given patient. Then, that information, combined with a detailed history of the patient, served as the basis for the formulation of an intervention plan. Ray's role in that plan was to choose or prescribe the combination of therapies most likely to yield the best health outcome based on the patient assessment. It was precisely that skill that helped give Ray his much-deserved reputation as a first-rate practitioner; he knew the importance of a good diagnosis and had the ability to strategically apply the combination of therapeutic tactics most likely to be effective.

Ray's thoughts shifted to his new situation. He was confident that he and his colleagues in the HAWC at Dobbins would be able to do the strategic planning part, but he was less certain about their ability to apply the right tactics to the right situation. Lela's chess story brought to light something Ray had perhaps unconsciously pushed into the shadows: Health promotion tactics or methods were something he needed to know much more about.

With that thought, Ray returned to his stack of readings. He finished the first article and turned to the next one, which had a handwritten note from Colonel Gayle stapled to the first page:

Ray:

Although this article is a few years old, I think it illustrates how multiple methods of health promotion can be applied to a single problem. I created a modification of the authors' table that we have used in some seminars and workshops—we have found the table a useful tool to help people see how the different attributes of various health promotion methods can be combined to create what we call a comprehensive approach. Hope it helps. See you in Atlanta.

Tim

Ray read the article. It had been published by Donald Reid and some of his fellow health promotion workers in England and described various intervention options that might be employed in a comprehensive tobacco-use prevention and control program at the national level.[1] The modified table that Colonel Gayle mentioned in his note was laid out in a matrix. The columns in the matrix represented criteria upon which any given health promotion tactic might be rated: effectiveness, reach, acceptability, cost, and public support. Each row listed different tactics. The cells of the matrix were blank, allowing planners to enter their assessment of how well a given tactic met each criterion. In all, there were five pages of matrices, each listing four to five different tactics in the row headings. On the first of these pages (Figure 6.1), four categories of tactics were listed: (1) health communication; (2) media advocacy; (3) policy, regulatory, and environmental actions; and (4) tailored communication.

Tactics	Effectiveness	Reach	Acceptability	Cost	Public Support
Health communication					
Media advocacy					
Policy, regulatory, and environmental actions					
Tailored communication					

Health Problem or Issue:_____

Objective:_____

FIGURE 6.1 Colonel Tim Gayle's Modification of the Reid et al. Table

Colonel Gayle had also attached a list of simple definitions, next to which he had written another note for Ray:

Ray:

Recently, we have carried out some in-service training on a variety of intervention "tactics" (e.g., school health, mass media, policy development). As a part of that training, we give participants "evidence" that will enable them to put information in the open cells of the matrix. Then we have them talk with their fellow participants and come to a consensus as to what information should go into each cell.

Tim

The definitions for each of the criteria listed in the column headings were listed below the table:

- **Effectiveness**—the extent to which there is evidence that this tactic, when properly applied, will contribute to attaining the objective for which it was chosen

- **Reach**—the potential for reaching a large proportion of the target audience
- **Acceptability**—the extent to which the target audience, general public, and relevant agencies find the tactic to be within the range of actions that are socially and culturally acceptable
- **Cost**—the extent to which the proper application of the tactic is economically feasible
- **Public Support**—the extent to which the effective application of a tactic has potential for engendering positive public opinion and, therefore, support for either the issue in particular or public health and prevention in general

Ray thought to himself how the matrix reminded him of a chess board.

Case Analysis

We don't know whether Captain Rodriguez got off the airplane with more insight about the job he was about to undertake than he had when he boarded a few hours earlier. However, we do know that the chess analogy reminded him that an effective intervention requires two complementary skills, both of which must be applied strategically: (1) the ability to carry out a sound analysis of the health problem and the multiple factors associated with that problem and (2) the knowledge and capacity to apply the methods or tactics most likely to effectively address that problem. The previous chapters in this book have attended primarily to issues related to the former set of skills; we now focus on the latter.

SIX PRINCIPLES

Over the years, we have had the pleasure of meeting and visiting with experienced health promotion practitioners from around the globe. In spite of language and cultural differences, we have observed that effective practitioners seem to act on six practical principles that serve as a mental model for selecting the tactics most likely to achieve their program objectives.

Principle 1: Use Objectives to Stay Focused

Not only do effective practitioners take seriously the task of identifying practical, specific, and measurable objectives, but they revisit those objectives often to make sure they are on track.[2] Recall our earlier reference to the children's pedestrian-injury prevention project in Perth, Australia; project staff had affixed a flow chart of their program plan, including specific intervention objectives, on their office wall. They found this simple technique to be an effective means to help them keep their intervention ideas focused on program objectives. (See Tables 4.1 and 4.2.)

Principle 2: Make Informed Decisions

Simply put, the probability that you will select methods and tactics that will work (i.e., achieve your program objectives) increases proportionately with your understanding of the people involved and the environment where the intervention will take place. All effective practitioners use some routine process to assess existing levels of knowledge, attitudes, capacities, and environmental supports. Their ultimate intervention decisions are shaped by their interpretation of the information they obtain from that process in light of behavioral, social, and learning theory.

Principle 3: Don't Reinvent the Wheel

Like accomplished athletes, experienced practitioners waste little "motion" because they know the wisdom of simplicity. For health promotion practitioners, simplicity begins with taking the time to see and confirm what the community already has to offer before trying to envision new intervention ideas. Often, fine-tuning an existing program will suffice and is likely to have the added benefit of demonstrating respect for prior efforts undertaken by the community.

Principle 4: There Is No Such Thing as a Free Lunch

We all know of creative practitioners who have used volunteers or have been able to secure a pro bono component for a given aspect of a health promotion program. But one must take care not to mistake these creative actions with the reality that it takes economic and human resources to implement and sustain a program over time. For experienced practitioners, the decision to select a given intervention method or tactic will in part be determined by the estimated costs of implementing that method.

We have found it helpful to think of three categories of costs: economic costs, time costs, and opportunity costs. Economic costs include such things as salaries and benefits, materials, equipment, printing, and media time. Time is a cost in the sense that it is a necessary commodity for planning and preparation; when planners do not allow sufficient time for preparation and coordination among sectors, they put their programs at risk for failure. Finally, when colleagues agree to lend you their personal support for your program, that means they have to give up or lower their level of effort on something else; this is an opportunity cost. Recall the case story of Linda Thomas in Chapter 1. Even though she held the stress management sessions during her own lunch time, the project absorbed her attention, energy, and at least some portion of her time. Thus, her decision to devote time to the stress reduction effort did have a cost in that it diminished and took away from the opportunity to invest her energy in another program.

Principle 5: To Maximize Effectiveness, Strategically Combine Multiple Tactics to Influence Complex Problems

Matrices such as the one illustrated in the "Checkmate" case story give us the kind of information needed to ensure that all of the key issues are being addressed, that we are taking a strategic and comprehensive approach. After an exhaustive review of the most effective environmental and policy tactics to reduce tobacco use, Brownson and his colleagues provided this wisdom about the importance of comprehensiveness:[3]

> Environmental and policy interventions may have greater impact
> if they are carried out over multiple settings—health care, schools,
> or worksites, in addition to the whole community (p. 480).

Principle 6: Be Creative

Media advocacy pioneer Mike Pertschuk once said this about his own specialty: "Media advocacy requires art, imagination, and creativity; any attempt to reduce it to a series of rigid and prescribed steps is doomed to mediocrity and failure." We agree with Pertschuk's sentiment and believe that it is a good reminder for the application of virtually all health promotion interventions. At the same time, however, this call for creativity should not be taken as a diminution of the importance of careful analysis, the application of theory, and sound management. On the contrary, creativity in public health is expressed by combining thoughtful judgment with the freedom to use one's imagination. As has been emphasized throughout this book, health promotion should not be expressed by the routinized application of a prescribed, one-size-fits-all "cookbook" program.

The remainder of this chapter is divided into two sections. The first section describes the five tactics that appeared on the first page of the matrix Ray received from Colonel Gayle: health communication; media advocacy; policy, regulatory, and environmental actions; and tailored communication (see Figure 6.1). The second section illustrates how multiple tactics can be combined to create a more "comprehensive" approach to addressing health promotion objectives.

HEALTH COMMUNICATION: FOLLOW THE SIGNPOSTS

What do you call it when you exchange thoughts and information with someone? Communication, of course! The Latin root for the word *communication* is *communicare,* meaning "to make common." As used in the context of public health and health promotion, the concept of health communication certainly incorporates the intuitive objective of making sound health information "common" among all people. It also incorporates another important element: analysis. By *analysis,* we mean the systematic examination and interpretation of information to make informed decisions—specifically, decisions about what messages to share, with whom to share them, what are the most efficient ways to share them, and what are the most appropriate channels through which to disseminate them. Without such systematic analysis, health communication efforts run the risk of being driven by opinions (which may not be true), anecdotes (which may not be typical), or stories (which may not be accurate).

Effective practitioners don't guess at the actions they should take; they make decisions. Their decisions are informed by their knowledge of what has gone on in the past and what is going on around them in the present. Effective practitioners are empowered to the extent that they have and use relevant information.

One simple key to taking a systematic approach to health communication is knowing which questions to ask. Based on selective doses of our own experiences and borrowing liberally from some of our favorite resources,[4] we offer the following sequence of health communication "signposts," framed as questions. In seeking responses to these common-sense questions, practitioners will generate most of the information they will need to make informed and insightful decisions.[5]

Signpost 1: What Can Health Communication Do for You?

As you consider the use of health communications, keep in mind that this approach, like all health promotion tactics, has its strengths and weaknesses.

Here are some things that health communication tactics can accomplish:

- Increase public awareness of a health issue, problem, or solution
- Stimulate individuals' reexamination of positive shifts in health-related attitudes
- Demonstrate or illustrate skills
- Bring to light key health issues to increase public demand for action on those issues
- Reinforce knowledge, attitudes, or behavior

Here are some things that health communication tactics are not likely to accomplish:

- Produce behavior change without supportive program components
- Be equally effective in addressing all issues or relaying all messages
- Compensate for a lack of essential staff

Suppose that you are involved in a breast cancer early-detection program. One of the key objectives of the program is to increase by 50 percent the number of women age 50 and older in your service area who have had a screening mammogram. The decision as to whether a given health communication tactic should be part of your overall intervention strategy will obviously be informed by data you have gathered in prior planning steps. This information could include the prevalence of screening mammograms among women over 50 by level of education, income, and locale; the attitudes of physicians regarding the importance of screening mammograms in their practices; and the perceptions of women about the risks, benefits, costs, availability, and accessibility of screening services. In combination, the next two signposts can help you decide which pieces of information are most relevant.

Signpost 2: With Whom Are You Trying to Communicate?

In the breast cancer screening example, the target group might be all women over 50, or the subset of women over 50 who have not had a mammogram. Alternatively, it might include husbands, friends, or family members of women over 50 who have not had a mammogram. It could also be primary-care physicians, owners of businesses in the service area that serve women over 50, or some combination of all of these.

In the language of market research, determining your specific audience is called segmenting the market. Once you have identified the audience (segment) to be reached, your probe for information continues with an audience analysis. In this process, you try to become aware of the characteristics you need to take into account if you are to make effective contact with the group in question.

Why is such analysis necessary? Because social marketing theory and empirical evidence confirm what common sense tells us: not everyone responds the same way to the same message.[6] Depending upon the diversity and size of the group, important characteristics might include age, sex, level of education, current level of awareness about (and attitudes toward) the problem, occupation, geographic location, and cultural orientation. Whether the group in question consists of Sudanese villagers at risk of infection from dracunculiasis (guinea worm disease) or influential business leaders with the power to change environmental policies, the need for specific information, and the process to obtain it, remains the same.

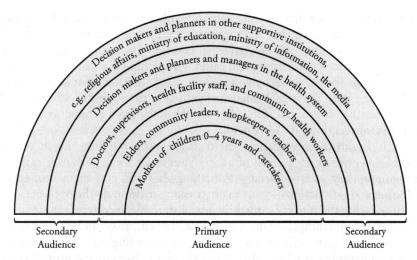

FIGURE 6.2   Primary and Secondary Audiences for Oral Rehydration

Some communications experts suggest that there is merit in dividing audiences into subgroups. For example, Figure 6.2 identifies five audiences who are relevant to a priority health problem in all developing countries: diarrheal disease.[7] Note that two groups (mothers and caretakers of children age zero to four; and community elders, leaders, shopkeepers, and teachers) have been designated as the primary audience and the remaining three groups as the secondary audiences. The positioning of the secondary audiences purposefully reflects their respective relationships with the primary audience. As such, it provides us with two graphic reminders:

1. We need to pay heed to secondary audiences because they can and often do function as channels of communication to other secondary audiences and to the primary audience. (See signpost 4 for additional details on channels of communication.)

2. In addition to the primary audience, secondary audiences may be a priority for communications attention. Consider the frontline staff and medical practitioners in the third-tier semicircle in Figure 6.2. Although they may be quite skilled in providing medical services, they may not perceive the merits of taking the time (or may lack the ability) to communicate the needs and benefits of oral rehydration therapy (ORT), proper feeding, and preventive practices to those they are serving.

Signpost 3: What Does It Cost Your Audience to Hear Your Message?

In consumer marketing, the price of a particular product is usually clear to both the customer and the marketer because it has a specific dollar value assigned to it—one that the consumer can either accept or reject. Of course, many factors affect whether a consumer will buy a particular product (hence the advertising industry!). Nevertheless, consumer transactions generally involve exchanging your hard-earned cash for something that you really want or need, or that someone has convinced you that you really want or need. The price (along with the inconvenience of getting to the store and other factors) represents the cost to you. Thus, the act of purchasing a product is a way of saying that you think it's worthwhile.

In health communication, the costs are much murkier, and so are the benefits or incentives. Instead of asking your audience to fork over cash for something they want or need—something that will give them immediate pleasure and satisfaction—you are often asking them to do the opposite. You may be asking them to try something uncomfortable, inconvenient, unfamiliar, and/or frightening, for which immediate benefits may not be apparent. In fact, the immediate effects may be quite discouraging! Quitting smoking, getting a mammogram, and changing one's diet or exercise patterns all come to mind as examples of health behaviors that can have a high sticker price for some audiences.

In analyzing your audience segments and designing your messages, make sure that you understand the "costs" that your audiences perceive. That understanding becomes the grounds upon which you can base messages to clarify misconceptions, allay fears, or both.

Signpost 4: What Do You Want to Say?

The task of determining with whom you want to communicate is virtually inseparable from the task of determining the most appropriate message to communicate. The goal here is to have a clear understanding of what the audience in question should do as a result of its exposure to your message. For example, in terms of your ultimate project goal, are you trying to achieve shifts among the audience in visiting health care providers, calling a hotline number, reading specific literature, using a certain product, or setting aside time to exercise?

Specificity is important in selecting a message. For example, urging a population of women in Los Angeles to "Get a mammogram," or a group of villagers in Ghana to "Drink clean water," may be too general. More specific messages, such as "Ask a health care provider whether you should have a mammogram" or "Drink water that has been passed through a proper filter," may be more realistic and appropriate.

Again, your initial ideas about the intent and content of the message will be informed by information gleaned during earlier planning. Once you have framed your initial idea for messages, social marketing research experts would encourage you to pretest those ideas to ensure that the audience for whom they are intended will see them as interesting, memorable, understandable, acceptable, relevant to their situation, and credible.

An excellent academic resource describing both the theory and methods of designing health messages is a book by that title: *Designing Health Messages,* edited by Maibach and Parrott.[8] It contains detailed accounts and many examples of message design and testing efforts. Included in this publication is a description by Lefebvre and his colleagues[9] of the research that went into the formulation of some of the messages in the "5 a Day for Better Health" program campaign carried out by the National Cancer Institute.[10] After acknowledging that the costs for original market research and analysis can be potentially prohibitive for large-scale campaigns, they explain how, by searching and analyzing data from secondary sources, they were able to obtain the information required to design effective messages at a much lower cost. For the "5 a Day" campaign, secondary sources included marketing databases that had been established and were periodically updated by various companies, associations, and organizations. We highlight this point to alert practitioners to the possibility that as the technology for creating and tracking consumer databases becomes more refined, such databases (at reasonable costs) are likely to become more widely available and readily accessible for health communication planning.

That said, most health promotion workers, especially those who serve in small or remote areas, will have to conduct their own customized message and materials testing, instead of relying on secondary sources. A variety of methods (singly or in combination) can be used to pretest messages and materials. These include questionnaires, focus groups, theater testing, central-location intercept interviews, and readability testing. A U.S. National Institutes of Health publication, *Making Health Communications Work: A Planner's Guide,* is a good source of background information on health communications, and contains very clear and practical descriptions of these basic pretesting methods.

Signpost 5: How Will the Message Get to Your Audience?

Generally, market researchers define the term *channel* simply as "the vehicle that transmits a message from a source to a receiver." Here are some examples of channels that community health promotion practitioners might consider:

- Interpersonal or face-to-face interaction (teacher to student, parent to child, physician to patient)
- Planned group meetings or gatherings (workplaces, communities of faith, classrooms)
- The community (libraries, periodic civic events, local government organizations, shopping centers and malls)
- Mass media (radio, television, newspapers, magazines, newsletters, direct mail, billboards)

- The Internet (electronic mail, Web pages, bulletin boards)
- Organizations or associations (volunteer health organizations, service organizations, professional societies)

Here are three basic questions to ask prior to making your choices about the channels most appropriate for your situation:

- Given the budgetary, personnel, and time resources available to you, is the channel feasible?
- Will the audience perceive this channel to be credible?
- Does the proposed channel fit the purpose of the health communication; that is, if your goal is to raise awareness of a new service, is there any evidence that use of this channel will work?

Earlier we defined *channel* as a vehicle through which a source sends a message to a receiver. Of course, sometimes the source (also referred to as the sender) and the channel are one and the same—for example, a parent communicating with a child, or vice versa, as in the case of school health programs that feature children communicating health ideas to their parents. We highlight this overlap to alert practitioners to the reality that a health communication effort is likely to be severely compromised if the receiver has doubts about or conflicts with the sender or source.

We found this statement to be true based on our effort to evaluate the American Cancer Society's Reach to Recovery Program.[11] Reach to Recovery is a service program wherein volunteers provide postsurgical support to women who have undergone surgery for breast cancer. The goal of the program is to assist patients in making a healthful adjustment to their surgery and to help them get on with normal lives. The volunteers in this program are women who themselves have experienced and made healthful adjustments to breast cancer surgery. The importance of the credibility of the volunteers in this program was best reflected in this quote from a patient in Pennsylvania:

> When a Reach volunteer walks into that hospital room, looking happy and balanced, she sends a message of hope to that patient— the kind of hope that neither the physician nor nurse can provide.

An important observation in this evaluation was that the credibility of having undergone the same experience (e.g., breast cancer surgery) was insufficient when there were cultural or ethnic differences between the volunteer and the patient. In addition, on-site interviews revealed that, in some instances, even the standard visit approach seemed to be incompatible. For example, it was reported that in one-on-one visits, Hispanic women in Los Angeles felt uncomfortable because they were asked to disclose intimate information to a "stranger." Further inquiry revealed that a "support group" approach in a place that the patient perceived as being friendly surroundings was much more acceptable.

Such accounts remind us not to lose sight of the common-sense courtesy inherent when you are consciously respectful of cultural differences. They also remind us why the community is the center of gravity for health promotion. Decisions about priorities and strategies for social change are best made as close as possible to where people work, live, and go to school. Communities are relevant, and it is precisely because community health promotion practitioners work amid such relevance that they have so much potential for making a difference.[12]

That said, the Australian health promotion expert Simon Chapman offers us this cautionary note about the inherent superiority of one approach over another:

> The top down or "done to" approach is frequently depicted as heinous and Stalinist, whereas "done with" approaches are seen as politically correct and mandatory. This dichotomy is far too simplistic: there are many examples where top down/done to/upstream strategies in health promotion (so-called passive prevention strategies), initiated by non-consulting health professionals, have been greeted warmly by the public and shown to have benefited public health in important ways. Random breath testing, comprehensive food labeling, Papanicolaou smears, mandatory bicycle crash helmets and vehicle seat belts, fluoridated water supply, taxes on cigarettes and alcohol, vehicle safety checks and standards . . . this list could go on. All these are hardly popular in the sense that they cause people to take to the streets, many involve things being "done to" people, many have been introduced with next to no involvement or loud expressions of interest by consumers, yet many of them are the success stories of modern public health.[13]

MEDIA ADVOCACY: ADDRESSING THE "MANUFACTURERS OF ILLNESS"

Recall that in Chapter 2, Archie Graham made reference to the classic study by Michael McGinnis and Bill Foege indicating that the "actual" causes of death are linked identifiable behavioral and environmental factors, all of which are amenable to change. Such analyses suggest that there is substantial public health merit in seeking to alert the public to the preventable nature of the leading causes of death. In the language of supply and demand, the main focus of this approach has been on the demand side: (1) strengthening the capacity (knowledge, healthful practices) of those at risk and (2) creating surroundings conducive to health. The health communication tactics described in the previous section are designed to address these important demand factors.

At the same time, clearly some of the important causes of today's priority health problems may fall outside the lens of our traditional epidemiologic focus. For example, although their role in ill health is well recognized by public health officials, corporations that produce tobacco, alcohol, handguns, and automatic weapons are not classified in terms of relative risk. These "manufacturers of illness" represent the supply side of the equation because they produce and aggressively market products with little or no regard for their negative effects on health.[14] Common sense tells us that a health promotion program aimed at the demand side but ignoring the supply side is bound to be weaker than a program that systematically addresses both. Doesn't it seem futile to teach youth about tobacco-, alcohol-, and drug-abuse prevention in a community where cigarettes, alcohol, and drugs can be purchased as easily as groceries? Does it make sense to withhold our efforts to inform and educate the public about healthful eating while we simultaneously undertake the long-range process of developing policies that will make low-fat dairy products available and accessible?

Enter Media Advocacy and Politics

We emphasize media advocacy precisely because its aim is to address the evasive, often political supply aspect of health problems. Practitioners should keep in mind the important distinction between health communication (social marketing) and media advocacy. Although both can employ the media, the former tends to promote personal responsibility and lifestyle change, while the latter seeks to attain the implementation of healthful policy.

The word *advocate* means "to defend, support, or champion a person or cause." It is a word that connotes passion and action. Although advocates are respectful of convention, it is not at all unusual for them to choose to support their cause over adherence to a convention. The advocacy approach differs in character from the standard practice of planning health promotion and disease prevention programs, which is grounded in epidemiology, the basic science of public health. Epidemiologic analysis gives us clues about the causal chain of events that lead to a particular health problem; in turn, this knowledge serves to guide us in the formulation of prevention and health promotion programs.

The Chapter 3 case story, "The Court of Public Opinion," made the point that public health work is political. Decisions are political whenever limited public resources will be distributed and those involved in the decision-making process do not agree about who should get what. For example, suppose you are a member of a community council, and the council members are responsible for annual budget decisions for all community services. Suppose further that you are convinced that the schools need a financial boost, but you are uncertain about the needs of four other departments: roads, police, parks and recreation, and public health. You are a sincere, hard-working, busy person, and you find little time for studying the many issues in front of you. Your support is sought by all of these groups. A trusted good friend of the family has encouraged you to take a special look at the business benefits that would occur if the parks and recreation department's lake revitalization project were funded. Can't you almost feel the political pull in that situation? The reality is that politics are ubiquitous. The challenge for the public health community in general, and for health promotion workers in particular, is to acknowledge that reality and to work efficiently and ethically within it.

Some Practical First Steps

Current health promotion literature offers rich and creative guidance on the implementation of media advocacy; we strongly urge practitioners to consult these existing resources for added depth and detail on the process.[15] In this section, we highlight a few practical issues that we hope will help practitioners get their teeth into media advocacy.

Larry Wallack and Lori Dorfman are public health professionals whose lucid writing and training efforts have done much to enhance our awareness and understanding of media advocacy.[16] To help give their audiences a sense of what media advocacy is about, they often use this quote attributed to Scoop Nisker, of KFOG radio in San Francisco: "If you don't like the news, go out and make some of your own!"

In effect, Nisker is saying several things here: (1) don't whine—it won't get you anywhere; (2) identify the "news" you want the public to attend to; and (3) take the initiative and action necessary to get the news to the public. *Media advocacy* refers to the use of mass media as a means of heightening the public's awareness of a problem and providing individuals with a means to take legitimate action to address that problem.

We have often thought that having media advocacy skills is like having access to a powerful searchlight that illuminates key unattended public health issues. Because the issues in question are often those that special interests may want to obscure or misrepresent, one important political result of bringing those issues into full public light is that decision makers are likely to feel uncomfortable if they ignore them.

As in undertaking any organized plan, it is important to be clear on what you want to accomplish. Following are three preliminary steps to help practitioners initiate a media advocacy effort.

Step 1: Identify Your Group's Policy Goal (What Do You Want to Happen?)

Suppose that the issue in question is youth violence. Your options might include the following:

- Limit handgun availability
- Limit alcohol availability
- Increase employment opportunities for youth

Key Point: Research your options carefully and be prepared to justify your policy actions for health improvement on the basis of empirical evidence.

Step 2: Identify Your Targets (To Whom Do You Want to Speak? When This Person, Group, or Organization Speaks, Will People Listen?)

In most health promotion interventions, the target audience consists of those persons at risk of developing a problem: teen smokers, women over age 50 who have not had a mammogram, children age five to ten who walk in a heavy traffic area. In media advocacy, there are three potential target audiences, listed here in descending order of importance: (1) a primary target consisting of the person or group with the power to make a policy change; (2) a secondary target consisting of individuals who can be mobilized to influence people or groups with the power to make the change; and (3) the general population.

Primary targets might include the following:

- The city council
- The mayor
- Business leaders

Secondary targets might include the following:

- Advocacy groups
- Professional societies
- Well-known, respected community leaders

Key Point: Be specific and stay focused on your target audience.

Step 3: Be Sure Your Message or Story Is Clear

All too frequently we hear that the media "just didn't get the story right!" While it is quite possible that they didn't, at least part of the problem can probably be attributed to a failure on the advocate's part to make the message or story clear. To help us sharpen the clarity of our message, Wallack and Dorfman ask us to pay particular attention to three elements of our communication with the media:

- **Be clear about the statement of concern.** "Tobacco is everywhere, and youth are especially at risk because . . ."
- **Highlight a value dimension.** "Tobacco companies are making economic profit with literally no regard to the unnecessary death, disease, and disability they cause."

- **Have unambiguous policy objectives.** "Stores that sell tobacco to minors will be fined $5000 per incident."

Key Point: Getting the media's attention is an important point, but don't stop there; have a specific message ready once you've gotten their attention! Be prepared to help members of the media write their script if asked.

Finally, throughout the process of planning a media advocacy effort, responsible practitioners will create a system for monitoring the progress and effects of all of these steps. Routine analysis and discussion of such information among members of your planning team are the most efficient means of assessing how you are progressing and, more importantly, what changes are necessary to keep you on course.

If You Don't "Frame It" Correctly, They Aren't Likely to Get It!

The effective application of media advocacy depends on a good understanding of the concept of framing. In this age of information, we can all identify with the struggle of having to sift through never-ending attempts to get our attention—e-mail, faxes, meetings, telephone solicitations, surveys, mailorder catalogs, newspaper headlines; the list seems endless. Obviously, what we attend to will depend on our perceived needs and interests—that is, we are likely to pay attention to information that is packaged, or framed, in a context that interests us. Wallack and Dorfman suggest that media advocacy is organized around two complementary frames: framing for access and framing for content. In both cases, the broad concept remains the same: package your information so that those for whom it is intended will pay attention.

Framing for Access

Framing for access means preparing your story in such a way that you maximize your chances of getting access to the media. If you took the time to make a listing of the stories covered on the local and network television and radio news programs, you would note that virtually all of the programs cover the same stories. Obtaining this kind of broad and repeated exposure for a critical health issue is a first-level objective of media advocacy.

As practitioners make plans to gain access to the media, the most fundamental idea we can offer is this: Think like a reporter. Make an appointment with a TV, radio, or newspaper reporter and simply ask some straightforward questions:

How do you gather news?

How do you determine which stories will be aired or printed?

What can I give you that will make your job easier?

Framing for Content

Framing for content means preparing a story in such a way that it prompts the target audience to acknowledge that any serious consideration of a solution to the problem must go beyond the individuals or victims involved, by including policy actions that can influence the environmental/social conditions that made the problem possible in the first place.

THE KEY: ANTICIPATION

Great athletes are also great anticipators. For example, effective shortstops in baseball anticipate that every ball will be hit to them. With full knowledge of the number of runners on base, the number of outs, the kind of pitch the pitcher plans to deliver, the speed of the runners, and the teams' defensive strengths and weaknesses, the shortstop calculates all of the possible contingencies before they occur. Because they are disciplined to anticipate, great athletes never seem to hesitate or give the appearance that they are in doubt. When asked why he always seemed to be in the right place at the right time, hockey star Wayne Gretzky replied simply, "I skate to where I think the puck will be!"

Practitioners whose mental model of health promotion includes media advocacy also anticipate well. They look for and scan stories and events for their advocacy potential—in fact, for the busy practitioner in the field, piggybacking, or tying your issue to a breaking news story, may constitute the best opportunity to attract news coverage. Editorial commentaries, letters to the editor, op-ed pieces, and talk show appearances can provide an effective and timely means for obtaining coverage.[17] Interviews with practitioners who have effectively applied media advocacy have inspired us to create the following scenario, followed by a series of circumstances and questions designed to stimulate your thinking about the options afforded you to get your message framed and "out there."

Scenario

For some time, you have been seeking policy action that addresses the fact that youth in Newbury have easy access to alcohol. Existing laws are not enforced.

Feature Story in the *Newbury News*

The citizens of Newbury today are mourning the death and serious injury of six teenagers from their community. Last night, six teenagers in a six-passenger sport-utility vehicle were returning from an early-evening party at Old Mountain. They had been celebrating their upcoming graduation from high school. There was dancing, singing, and volleyball at the party—and there was also plenty of cold beer. All of the passengers in the car had been drinking, including the driver. Eyewitnesses in the car behind the victims indicated that it appeared as if the driver lost control of his car on a sharp turn and hit a tree near the roadside. Two of the teenagers were killed and four were injured, three seriously. [Initially, the media frame this story around the notion that teens and parents need to take more responsibility to prevent alcohol-related problems.]

Situation 1

Knowing that you work on this issue, a reporter from the Newbury paper contacts you and asks for your comment. What do you say?

- Do you have a prepared statement?
- Do you have a list of reputable, credible local resource people who are willing to help make and support your point of view?
- Do you have to clear your comments to the media through your supervisor, the agency public relations office, or your agency director?
- Are you prepared to point to successful policy actions that other communities have taken to address this issue?

Situation 2

Members of the media contact you specifically to comment on (you suspect they would like you to support) their contention that this event is yet another example of the deterioration of family responsibility. What do you say?

- Did you anticipate this kind of confirmation request, and are you prepared to frame your response to get your message across?
- Are you prepared to refer them to reputable citizens who are willing to help make and support your point of view?

Situation 3

Members of the media contact your agency director for a comment. Did you anticipate your director being called?

- Did you brief your director in advance and leave him or her some written backup material?
- Does your director understand that he or she is not alone in the position you are advocating?

Situation 4

Members of the media don't call you, your director, or any of your colleagues. Consequently, the initiative for making contact with the media about this story shifts to you.

- Prior to this story breaking, did you take the time to establish prior relationships with members of the media?

- Have you obtained the appropriate clearance to make contact with the media?

- Have you prepared a written account that "frames" the story around the issues of youth access to alcohol?

POLICY, REGULATORY, AND ENVIRONMENTAL ACTIONS

The integration of policy, regulatory, and environmental actions into a health promotion program will strengthen that program in two ways. First, it declares that the issue in question is so important that it merits formal policy or regulatory support. The second benefit is that of longevity—that is, policy is as difficult to change as it is to implement. Therefore, once policies and environmental changes are in place, the chances of sustaining your health promotion initiative over time are increased. In this section, we will first illustrate the tactics of policy and regulatory action with an example from recent tobacco control efforts, then we will discuss environmental interventions more broadly at the close of the chapter.

Policy and Regulatory Actions

Because they can directly affect demand for and access to tobacco, legislative/policy tactics are among the most powerful tools that health promotion practitioners can employ in their efforts to control tobacco use. In addition, evidence suggests that, even when used as an independent action, legislative/policy tactics can significantly reduce tobacco consumption.[18]

However, the use of policy-oriented tactics is a complex and demanding undertaking. It requires careful orchestration and management of a well-organized, well-informed coalition whose membership is both politically savvy and patient. Practitioners must also be prepared for the very real possibility of backlash from those who feel that legislative actions infringe upon their freedom. In this section, we illustrate how six specific policy-oriented tactics can be orchestrated in combination to help practitioners attain a goal of reducing youth access to tobacco.

To begin with, you will find it useful to ask a series of questions to establish the climate for legislative action within your community. Such questions might include the following:

1. Have you identified individuals/organizations that could be advocates for tobacco-use control among youth?

2. Have you identified existing legislation regarding tobacco access to minors and retail tobacco license laws? Is this legislation enforced?

3. Have you identified a legislative outcome that you would like to see occur?

4. Are youth targeted within your community? Are any tobacco billboards located within 1000 feet of your schools?

Tactic A: Establish the Basic Groundwork

Recommended Actions

1. Conduct tobacco purchase surveys to determine the extent and magnitude of the problem within your community.

2. Obtain information on how and where minors get tobacco in your community or surrounding areas.

3. Prepare information that clearly describes the nature of the problem; use informal group testing to determine the extent to which citizens find the information you have prepared to be understandable and worth their attention.

Tactic B: Modify the Selling Practices of Merchants

Recommended Actions

1. As a first step, use existing communication channels to inform merchants, civic groups, and all relevant community organizations about the problem, emphasizing where and how youth get tobacco.

2. Encourage the local media to cover the problem of easy access to an addictive agent.

3. Conduct a merchant education program. Use a balanced approach, emphasizing civic responsibility and community benefits as well as the potential for penalties to owners, license suspension, and legal precedents for civil lawsuits against those in violation of sales-to-minors laws.

4. Create and post clever warning signs at all points of purchase.

5. Identify merchants whose practice it is not to sell tobacco to minors and make this information widely known as a healthful establishment (an honor similar to the Good Housekeeping seal of approval).

6. Identify merchants who do sell tobacco to minors and make this information widely known.

7. Promote the positive use of ID checks for all tobacco sales.

Tactic C: Increase Enforcement of Existing Laws Prohibiting Sales to Minors

Recommended Actions

1. If law enforcement agencies in your community do not consider enforcement of youth access laws to be a priority, explore the possibility of having

an alternative agency so designated—the public health department, for example.

2. Create a legitimate mechanism for citizens to file complaints against non-compliant merchants.

3. Create compliance checks and undercover buying operations (UBOs). These programs feature underage inspectors, accompanied by adult chaperons, who attempt to purchase tobacco products. UBOs do not result in any penalty to merchants, but rather demonstrate the extent of the problem, warn merchants, and constitute a very real precursor to enforcement.

4. Organize a community coalition to put pressure (through a public demonstration or the media) on relevant authorities to strengthen their enforcement practices.

5. Persuade law enforcement agencies to consider a "three strikes and you're out" policy for retail stores that consistently violate retail license laws and sales-to-minors laws. If enacted, this policy would mean that after three confirmed violations, retailers would have their licenses revoked or face other serious penalties.

6. Promote policies and community standards that prohibit the positioning of tobacco in easy-access places, such as in vending machines or on countertops in retail stores. In communities where this practice is illegal, establish fines and penalties for those establishments that continue to sell tobacco products to minors through vending machines.

7. Establish a standard coalition procedure in which members of your tobacco-use control coalition routinely communicate with politicians so as to remain informed about tobacco legislation as well as to inform the politicians about your views and goals.

Tactic D: Oppose Tobacco Advertising

More than 400,000 people die each year from tobacco-related causes;[19] 1.5 million more Americans quit smoking each year. To maintain its market, therefore, the tobacco industry must attract 2 million new smokers each year. Youth have been particularly vulnerable to tobacco advertising and promotion. Additionally, the tobacco industry specifically targets ethnic groups and women. Tobacco companies contribute extensively to political, social, and artistic organizations such as the Congressional Black Caucus, the National Women's Political Caucus, the Kool Jazz Festival, and Cinco de Mayo celebrations.

A well-known example of marketing specifically to a particular group was the 1989 attempt by the R. J. Reynolds Company to introduce Uptown cigarettes to African Americans as a niche market. At that time, menthol cigarettes (Newport, Kool, and Salem) were preferred by approximately three-fourths of black smokers.[20] Although Salem ranked as the fifth-best-selling brand in the industry and the best-selling menthol cigarette overall, its market share had been dropping because its strength was among white menthol smokers, a portion of the market that was declining.[21] The test market for the introduction of Uptown cigarettes was Philadelphia.

In a carefully documented account of the now famous Uptown incident, Sutton describes how a grass-roots community coalition successfully fought this test-marketing effort, resulting in R. J. Reynolds having to abandon its test marketing and, as a consequence, the entire Uptown strategy.[22] Sutton's detailed analysis provides very practical guidelines for carrying out a comprehensive approach to resisting corporate activities that are hazardous to health. She reminds us that those who direct such efforts would be well advised not to lose sight of the assets they have in the form of existing traditions and history.

> In prior community-based efforts in Philadelphia, the major communications mechanism used to rally the community to action had been the pulpit of the Black Church, not the news media. Therefore, the involvement of the Black Clergy of Philadelphia and a visibility of a Black minister as a key Coalition spokesperson was a critical in obtaining community support. The willingness of the Black Clergy to endorse the Coalition Against Uptown Cigarettes added to the credibility of the campaign and guaranteed a grassroots communications vehicle—Sunday services (p. 3).

Other, similar examples are widely documented in the health literature. For example, women's groups were enraged when the tobacco industry introduced Dakota cigarettes, which targeted young "virile" females. In many U.S. cities, billboards are disproportionately present in disadvantaged neighborhoods, and in the past, tobacco advertising predominated these billboards.[23]

Because billboard advertising of tobacco products is now prohibited in the U.S., tobacco companies rely more on other promotional strategies. Thus, before taking action, consider how you might address:

- event sponsorship by tobacco companies (e.g., music concerts, sporting events)
- free product samples
- advertising in alternative and special population media
- product placement in entertainment media

Recommended Actions

1. Orchestrate a campaign calling for the following:

   - A ban on the distribution of free tobacco samples or coupons for free samples through the mail or on property accessible to the general public

- A ban on tobacco advertising on public transit vehicles and in airports, train stations, and bus shelters

2. Write a sample policy that prohibits tobacco advertising in public facilities such as fairgrounds and sports facilities.

3. Lobby public officials to create smoke-free zones in public areas (such as airports, restaurants, and train stations).

4. Encourage citizens not to patronize facilities using tobacco advertising. (For example, a tobacco-use control coalition in California pressured county fair organizers to drop Phillip Morris as a sponsor. After the issue was widely covered by the media, the fair's board prohibited Marlboro-related promotional activities, and Phillip Morris pulled out as a sponsor.)

5. Lobby public officials to promote mandatory counteradvertising legislation.

6. Encourage public officials to eliminate the tax deductibility of tobacco advertising expenses.

7. Pressure legislators to enforce existing advertising laws (if any). Document violations of existing laws and failure to enforce those laws.

8. Strive for the removal of all tobacco advertisements within 1000 feet of a school.

9. Encourage alternative sponsorship of athletic, artistic, cultural, or musical events.

10. Lobby for legislation that reduces the number of tobacco advertisements or that ensures as many healthy messages as tobacco advertisements.

How to Lobby for Change

1. Communicate with or educate decision makers and the general public about the importance of tobacco-use control policies.

2. Advocate for specific policies considered by nonlegislative groups (e.g., school boards, state boards of health).

3. Advocate among audiences such as state attorneys general, regulatory authorities, or police authorities for more effective law enforcement or regulation.

4. Aim advocacy actions at government executives (such as mayors and governors).

5. Find out death rates due to coronary heart disease, lung cancer, and bronchitis in your community. Contact local cancer registries or birth/death registries.

6. Find out the prevalence of smoking in your community.

7. Call your legislators and ask what they plan to do about the preventable deaths that are occurring in their districts. They're losing valuable voters!

Effective lobbying is made up of the following components:

- A legislative liaison with the coalition
- Willing legislators
- An organized strategy
- A focused message
- A supportive coalition
- Legislative briefings
- Local events for legislators
- Press development

Tactic E: Offer Economic Incentives

Recommended Actions

1. Build a coalition to support raising the cigarette excise tax.
2. Change insurance policies to reward nonsmokers by:

   - Meeting with local business representatives to urge them to provide nonsmoker discounts for employees
   - Meeting with local insurance companies to request that they offer reimbursement for smoking-cessation programs

3. Encourage boycotts of nontobacco products produced by tobacco companies such as RJR Nabisco (e.g., Oreo cookies and other food products).

Tactic F: Look First for Existing Local Assets

All of the tactics described previously have been "field tested" and, to varying degrees, shown to lead to desirable health objectives and outcomes. As processes like these continue to emerge, the process and methodology become more refined—in short, we learn more and become better at doing it! As the new knowledge and learning proves valuable, it becomes more formalized in books and training programs, and sometimes triggers the emergence of new institutions. Such is the case with the National Association of African Americans for Positive Imagery (NAAAPI)—pronounced "nappy." The impetus for the formation of NAAAPI came primarily from the lessons learned from the historic defeat of Uptown cigarettes. The founders of NAAAPI wanted to use what they had learned to help end the excessive marketing of alcohol, tobacco, and other harmful products in communities of color.

NAAAPI's goal is to mobilize African American communities around the nation to support media and advertising images that are positive and healthy. The mission is to mobilize community members to live a healthy lifestyle, promote positive imagery in communities and among individuals, and foster environments free of health disparities. Since its inception, NAAAPI has played a role in health victories involving the removal of two other products that were marketed to African American youth: PowerMaster Malt Liquor in 1993 and X cigarettes in 1995. Group members have also mobilized against the introduction of Marlboro Milds, a menthol brand, and underage drinking in African American communities.

Organizations like NAAAPI are emerging around the world. We urge health promotion practitioners to look carefully within their local communities, or in those close by, for organizations with the experience in taking policy, political, and/or environmental actions to improve health.

Environmental Interventions

For many important health problems, environmental interventions go hand-in-hand with policy and regulatory actions. Environmental approaches are especially important as a complement to more frequently used behavioral and lifestyle tactics because they can benefit all people exposed to the environment rather than focusing on changing the behavior of one person at a time.[24]

Environmental interventions seek to change the conditions in which people live and may focus on the physical environment, the social environment, or both. The *physical environment* includes existing or potential community structures that may influence health behaviors and decisions. For example, some airports have recently built "smoking rooms" with separate ventilation systems. Within the airport, these rooms are the only place where travelers are permitted to smoke. The *social environment* includes a wide range of factors, from social norms to laws and policies. Continuing with the example of smoking in airports, policies prohibiting smoking in airport terminals, restaurants, restrooms, and on-board airplanes are all examples of policy actions in the realm of the social environment.

We are hard pressed to think of any health issue addressed by health promotion that would not benefit from a careful assessment of, and intervention upon, the environmental determinants of that problem. Consider some of the following examples:

- No matter how motivated individuals might be to exercise, it will be much more difficult to act on that motivation if the places to exercise are limited, difficult to access, or not safe.

- In response to the epidemic of obesity among children in the United States health promotion practitioners are actively encouraging kids to eat healthier foods and get more physical activity. Yet each day, millions of children who live close enough to walk to school don't do so. The reasons are complex, but certainly include aspects of the physical and social environment such as traffic and safety that can be major deterrents to children walking to school.

- National guidelines recommend that all Americans eat five to nine servings of fruits and vegetables each day, and keep their fat intake below 30 percent of total calories. Yet in many large U.S. cities, and especially those with significant low-income and minority populations, supermarkets are few and far between. The bodegas and convenience stores that do operate in these locations rarely offer a variety of healthy food choices and seldom stock fresh fruits and vegetables.

- Many skin cancers are largely a result of excessive exposure to ultraviolet (UV) light during childhood. Day-care centers and schools can help reduce children's risk by limiting recess time during peak UV hours (i.e., altering the social environment) and/or providing areas of shade on playgrounds (i.e., altering the physical environment).

- Injuries resulting from bicycle–automobile collisions are frequently quite serious. The most common health promotion response to this problem has been to encourage helmet use among cyclists. A less common, but perhaps equally important tactic is to provide separate spaces on roadways for autos and bikes. Adding bike lanes to heavily trafficked roads used by cyclists is an environmental intervention.

- Asthma affects about 8 to 12 percent of all children and 7 million adults in the United States, costing an estimated $6.2 billion per year. It is the most common chronic disease of childhood and a leading cause of disability among children. Many houses, but especially those in low-income areas, have problems with cockroaches. It is well documented that "roach dust"—roach body parts and roach droppings—is a very powerful allergen that "triggers" asthma attacks. Furthermore, evidence suggests that if children encounter fewer allergens early in life, they'll be less likely to develop allergic responses later on. A strategy to prevent and control asthma that *does not* include tactics to eliminate cockroaches and other sources of allergens known to trigger asthma attacks will be incomplete.

Reminders or "Prompts"

The following steps are offered as "prompts" to encourage practitioners to look for opportunities to incorporate environmental intervention tactics as a part of their health promotion strategy:

1. When using the assessment methods described in Chapter 4, carefully document the environmental factors that influence the health problem

directly as well as the environmental factors that directly influence the health behaviors associated with the health problem.

2. Environmental interventions often require political approval/or significant financial resources. Therefore, practitioners may find it helpful to consider the following questions as they assess the changeability of environmental factors:

   • Does the environmental action you are proposing require government approval, such as zoning, licensure, or construction standards? Who among those whose approval is needed is most likely to be in favor of (and opposed to) the action?

   • What, if any, resources will be needed to enact the environmental change? What do these resources cost? Can allies in the community donate or provide needed resources and services at a reduced cost?

3. Once you have identified critical environmental factors and determined that they are important and changeable, look for (through your past experience, network of colleagues, or the literature) communities that have successfully put in place tactics to redress similar environmental issues. If possible, contact them and ask whether they could share their experiences and suggestions.

Be Ready to Use "Evidence"

Where possible, use "evidenced-based" tactics. In the asthma example mentioned earlier, consider the challenge of developing tactics to eliminate cockroaches. Based on intuition, pesticide sprays, foggers, and bombs have been used for years to control cockroaches. Truth is, they don't work! They drive the roaches away for a while, only to have them return later. Furthermore, many of these chemicals leave too much residue either in the air or on household objects and, in fact, have been found to trigger asthma attacks.

Research (evidence) suggests that a more effective environmental approach, referred to as integrated pest management (IPM), keeps roaches away for good. Instead of pesticide sprays, it calls for the use of boric acid and roach baits as necessary. A key element in the IPM method is to deny roaches food, water, and shelter. Specific, evidenced-based environmental actions would include the following:

   • Cleaning up clutter such as piles of newspaper and clothing

   • Discarding grocery bags, cartons, boxes, and other containers that may bring roaches and roach eggs in from the outside and provide hiding places

   • Using a caulk gun to seal cracks and holes around baseboards, shelves, cupboards, pipes, sinks, and bathtub fixtures

- Spraying foam to fill holes, openings, and electric outlet boxes where roaches like to hide
- Making plastering repairs where there are large holes or damaged walls

While your first course of action should be to apply tactics shown previously to be effective, don't be afraid to take the wise counsel of Mike Pertschuk cited earlier in this chapter. That is, use your *imagination* and *creativity* to envision a new environmental intervention tactic. Creative thinking, backed by good assessment information, supported with input from stakeholders, and monitored with sound evaluation, is the key to effective innovations.

TAILORING: COMBINING TECHNOLOGY WITH THEORY

What Is Tailoring?

Have you ever bought a pair of shoes that seemed to fit in the store, but led to excruciating pain once you tried to walk around in them for a few hours? What about shoes that always give you a blister on one toe? And how often do you buy a pair of shoes by mail, without trying them on?

When you stop to think about it, shoes are an unlikely product to make in mass quantities, despite the many varieties available to us. After all, our feet are all a little bit different—different sizes, shapes, arches, toes, and widths. A particular size in one brand may not be exactly right in another brand. For some of us, our two feet aren't even exactly the same size! In fact, we would all be a lot more comfortable if we could afford custom-made shoes. Unfortunately, this is a luxury most of us will never enjoy. Just for a moment, though, imagine what it would be like.

Imagine walking into a shoe store. Instead of browsing for some mix of color, shape, and price (and desperately trying to get a salesperson's attention), you would walk up to a computer with a weird foot-shaped pad attached to it. You would step on the pad and let the computer measure every nuance of your foot—not only its length and width, but also the height of your arch, where the ball of your foot falls, the narrowness of your heel, where your ankle bone falls . . . perhaps even whether your feet sweat! Then you might answer a few questions about the color and style you are seeking and approve the price, and—voilá!—a perfectly fitted pair of shoes would be yours.

Futuristic fantasy? Maybe. But a similar approach is being used today in health promotion: using computerized interaction to "tailor" a health promotion program to the unique characteristics of the person for whom it is intended. We have chosen to highlight tailoring for two reasons: (1) it is a methodological approach that is gaining considerable interest as a means to deliver health education/promotion within the context of managed care, and

(2) it offers a clear, unambiguous illustration of how social, psychological, behavioral, and educational theory is applied in practice.

Health promotion materials are tailored when they are designed in any combination of strategies to reach one specific person and are (1) based on characteristics unique to that person, (2) related to the outcome of interest, and (3) derived from an individual assessment. This concept of trying to get a better "fit" is grounded in theory[25] and supported by a growing literature reporting encouraging effects.[26] But just as the costs of tailored clothes and shoes put them out of reach for most people, so the opportunity costs of tailoring health messages have traditionally caused many community health promotion practitioners to consider the process as having limited potential for reaching large numbers of people. In recent years, however, the application of computer technology in health promotion has changed that perception.

Tailoring Works!

Studies have shown that assessment-based, computer-generated materials that are tailored to the unique needs and interests of individual subjects can be effective for encouraging a variety of health-related behaviors, including smoking cessation,[27] dietary management,[28] obtaining screening mammograms,[29] and childhood immunizations. In these studies, subjects who received tailored behavior-change information were significantly more likely to make lifestyle changes than were those who received the usual medical care, untailored materials, or no messages.

Although tailoring, targeting, and personalizing are all associated with the notion of specificity, they are not synonymous. For example, earlier in this chapter we indicated that materials and messages could be targeted based on principles of market segmentation, which seek to identify key demographic characteristics of subgroups within the general population. Properly planned, this approach can lead to the development of educational materials that are more likely to be attended by the target populations; those materials would not be considered tailored, however.

Tailored health promotion materials also should not be confused with personalized materials. Personalization involves the use of a person's name to draw attention to an untailored message. A common commercial marketing example in the United States is the use of direct-mail tactics for the promotion of popular magazine sales (e.g., "Mary Beth Johnson, you may have already won $2,500,000!").

Both targeted and personalized communications base their messages on demographic factors such as age, race, sex, and name—all of which are unique to the potential receivers of the information. However, the assumption in tailoring is that demographic factors alone are not likely to provide the information sufficient to address complex health behaviors. For example, if you were developing a dietary-change program, which would be more useful to you—knowing the age, race, and sex of participants, or knowing about their specific dietary attitudes, habits, and eating patterns? A computerized tailoring approach enables you to draw on the strengths of both sources of information. In addition, the application of computer technology lessens the interview burden for the practitioner and the individual.

Tailored communication is grounded in the following assumptions:

- Individual assessment tends to eliminate superfluous information and bring into focus information that is personally relevant to the recipient.

- People pay more attention to information they perceive to be personally relevant.

- Information that draws one's attention is more likely to stimulate or support action than information that does not.

How Are Tailored Materials Created?

The process of creating tailored health promotion materials involves five general tasks:

1. Analyzing the problem and understanding its determinants
2. Developing an assessment tool to measure a person's status based on these determinants
3. Creating tailored messages that address the determinants of the problem
4. Developing a database to store participants' responses
5. Developing tailoring algorithms that translate participants' responses from the database into tailored messages

Table 6.1 summarizes the major steps in carrying out these tasks. To act on these steps, health practitioners will need to call on their basic health promotion competencies in behavioral science theory, questionnaire design, and development of educational messages, and combine them with the skills of those capable of creating linked databases and general computer programming.[30] As our main purpose in highlighting the process of tailoring is to illustrate how theory directly affects the practitioner's selection of methods, we will focus our attention on the first three steps in the process. The endnotes[31] describe some of the key points of Steps 4 and 5. This description may pique the interest of students and practitioners with an eye for combining research and technology.

Step 1: Analyze the Problem

As we have emphasized throughout this book (but especially in Chapter 3), effective practitioners make it a priority to understand the determinants of

TABLE 6.1   Steps in Carrying Out the Key Tasks for Tailoring Health Promotional Materials

Analyzing the Problem	Developing an Assessment Tool	Creating Tailored Messages
1. Define the problem and target population 2. Identify factors that influence the problem (i.e., determinants) 3. Determine which of these factors are amenable to change 4. Prioritize among candidate determinants (i.e., select variables to be addressed in tailored communication) 5. Set objectives to be achieved by tailored communication	1. Identify or develop questions to measure key determinants 2. Identify potential response choices for each question 3. Prioritize among candidate response choices 4. Determine the best method for data collection 5. Pretest the assessment tool among members of the target population	1. List assessment questions and response choices to be addressed by tailored messages 2. Identify intervention strategies that could be used to address each possible response choice for each assessment question 3. Determine which strategies can be delivered effectively via tailored messages 4. Develop message concepts describing how each strategy could be communicated in tailored messages 5. Pretest message concepts 6. Create tailored messages that address key message concepts 7. Pretest tailored messages

Developing a Database	Developing Tailoring Algorithms
1. Assign a variable name to each question in the assessment tool 2. Create a variable key that assigns a numeric value to each response choice for each question in the assessment tool 3. Develop a database to store respondents' answers to the assessment questions	1. Create a single message library that contains all tailored messages 2. Assign a different variable name to each tailored message in the library 3. Using the variable names from the questions and tailored messages, write "if/then" logic statements linking the numeric value of each response choice to its corresponding tailored message from the tailoring library 4. Incorporate algorithms into a single computer program that will merge participant responses from the database with messages from the tailoring library 5. Test the tailoring program extensively

the problem they seek to address. Consider again the metaphor of tailored messages being like custom-made shoes. For a shoemaker, the key measurements will vary depending on the type of shoe and the customer's measurements. Elegant fabrics, lines, and shapes might be required for dress shoes, while durability and comfort are required for sports shoes. The same is true for tailoring health promotion materials; the key "measurements," or determinants, vary depending on the outcome of interest. For example, a tailored program to help participants quit smoking may require an assessment of their readiness to quit[32] or their self-efficacy for quitting.[33] In contrast, tailored materials promoting breast cancer screening might focus on a woman's perceived risk of breast cancer, her beliefs about mammography, and the barriers to getting a mammogram that she perceives.

So how do you determine the key variables for a given health problem? First, get familiar with what you already know. Review the research literature describing the factors associated with the promotion of healthful behaviors; this search will generate ideas about the determinants to watch for. Globally, the health promotion research literature is a huge information resource, and it is getting better every year. As you scan the literature, see how prominent theories of health-related behavior change previously cited (e.g., the Transtheoretical Model, the Health Belief Model, self-efficacy and social learning theories) are used to explain the change process. To help you put all of this information into a manageable framework, we suggest that you use the process of identifying the causes described in Chapter 4.

This process will yield a list of candidate factors to be considered as key determinants of the outcome of interest. To narrow the list, consider which factors are most changeable, most important (i.e., have the greatest influence on the outcome of interest), and most pertinent for the particular population being addressed. Tailored interventions will be most efficient when this process identifies the fewest number of determinants that predict the greatest amount of change in the outcome of interest. As an example, analyzing the problem of cigarette smoking might reveal the following factors to be important for the outcome of cessation: readiness to quit, level of addiction to nicotine, perceived barriers to quitting, self-efficacy for quitting, motives for quitting, and past experience trying to quit.

Step 2: Develop an Assessment Tool

Because tailored materials are assessment-based, a questionnaire or survey must be developed to measure a person's status on each of the factors identified in Step 1. These surveys may be self-administered, administered by an interviewer, or even administered by an interactive computer program. Whatever the format, their distinguishing characteristic is a limited choice of answers. To create all possible tailored messages before the assessment takes place, the response choices to each question must be known. A major part of developing the assessment tool, then, is determining which response choices will accompany each assessment question.

To enhance efficiency, it will be most helpful if you use the smallest number of response options that are likely to capture the largest percentage of respondents. For example, if 100 smokers were surveyed, they might give 15 different reasons for wanting to quit smoking. If 90 of the smokers give one of five reasons, and each of the remaining 10 gives an entirely different reason, however, it is probably most practical for your question about motivation to quit to include just the five most common answers. But how do you identify the appropriate or most common response choices?

Research papers on the topic of interest present such data, as do review articles that summarize existing knowledge about changing a given behavior. In many cases, especially with theoretical variables, questions with established psychometric properties already exist and can be either used as is or modified to meet the needs of the tailoring assessment.

Building on the example from Step 1, responses to an assessment tool for smoking would yield valuable and specific information on such factors as readiness to quit, level of addiction to nicotine, perceived barriers to quitting, motives for quitting, self-efficacy for quitting, past experience trying to quit, and social support. Figure 6.3 provides an example of how responses to these seven factors create an individual profile—you can see that this level of information would be crucial to tailoring smoking-cessation programs and in communicating their robustness to others.

Step 3: Create Tailored Messages

When you have identified the key determinants of the outcome of interest, the questions to assess those determinants, and the most common response choices for each question, you will have the information necessary to begin crafting your tailored messages. Recall the references to mental models in earlier chapters. The mental model that guides the process of creating tailored messages provides us with an unambiguous illustration of how theory is used to inform the development of an intervention strategy and, therefore, the tactics needed to carry out that strategy.

Figure 6.4 offers a simple illustration of that process; let's walk through an example to see how it works. Suppose the goal is to provide tailored messages designed to increase physical activity among a population of senior citizens, as might be the case in either a senior citizens' center or a medical practice specializing in geriatrics.

The individuals in question are asked to complete a questionnaire. Each question is grounded in some aspect of theory deemed to be relevant to the goal. For example, consider the following questions:

Yes	No	Not Sure	
☐	☐	☐	Are you interested in improving your level of physical fitness?

Yes	No	Not Sure	
☐	☐	☐	Are you interested in improving your flexibility?

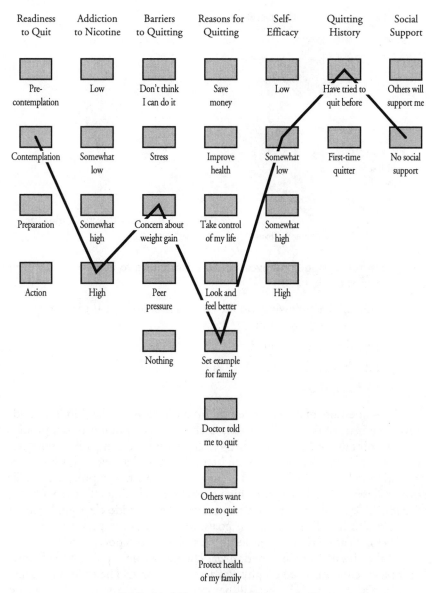

Readiness to Quit	Addiction to Nicotine	Barriers to Quitting	Reasons for Quitting	Self-Efficacy	Quitting History	Social Support
Pre-contemplation	Low	Don't think I can do it	Save money	Low	Have tried to quit before	Others will support me
Contemplation	Somewhat low	Stress	Improve health	Somewhat low	First-time quitter	No social support
Preparation	Somewhat high	Concern about weight gain	Take control of my life	Somewhat high		
Action	High	Peer pressure	Look and feel better	High		
		Nothing	Set example for family			
			Doctor told me to quit			
			Others want me to quit			
			Protect health of my family			

FIGURE 6.3   Individual Profile Generated from a Theory-Based Survey

A "Yes" response to these questions would suggest that the respondent is at the contemplation or ready-for-action stage, based on the Stages of Change theory. Not only does this answer give the planner important information about the individual's readiness for change, but it also provides insight into the strategies most likely to be attended to and tried by the respondent. A "Yes" response would also prompt the respondent to answer

Responses to Theory-Based Questions

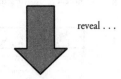

reveal . . .

Strategies for Change

which serve as
the basis for . . .

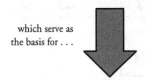

Messages to Promote Change

FIGURE 6.4   How Theory Guides the Tailoring Process

other questions designed to reveal added information to help in the decision process. For example:

> Which of the following would be a barrier to you initiating a physical activity program?
>
> a. I tried before and failed.
>
> b. I don't have the time.
>
> c. It's too difficult.

This question, of course, is derived from the Health Belief Model and addresses the issue of perceived barriers. Each response option acts as a prompt that will point in the direction of theoretically sound and compatible strategies. For example, if the "I tried before and failed" option was selected, sound theory, supported by research evidence, suggests that a strategy promoting skills associated with self-efficacy has a high probability of being effective with this individual. Based on this rationale, messages that provide clear guidance on how to establish realistic, attainable goals, ways to monitor personal progress, and tips for creating positive self-feedback would all be appropriate.

If the "It's too difficult" option was chosen, it might prompt the following message concept based on physical activity research: The maximum benefit in cardio-respiratory fitness will be obtained by moving from little or no physical activity to moderate levels, rather than from moderate to high levels.

The next step might be to test the effectiveness of such messages as "Just get moving" or "Walk, don't run!"

COORDINATE MULTIPLE TACTICS

We have described a selection of individual tactics that constitute part of what may be considered the health promotion practitioner's repertoire of methods. The art of health promotion practice lies not in the practitioner's ability to select a *single* tactic, but rather in his or her ability to integrate *multiple* tactics seamlessly into a coordinated effort to meet a single objective. Consider how the tactics described previously might be combined to help promote physical activity in community settings.

Suppose that in a given community health promotion practitioners working closely with community residents have identified sedentary lifestyle and its consequences as a major threat to quality of life in the community. Specifically, residents have expressed frustration that no safe, convenient, and pleasant places to exercise in town exist. They think that if such places existed, people in the community would use them. Some residents have heard that people in a neighboring town have built their own walking trail and that it is getting a lot of use. They like that idea and want to try it themselves in their own town.

As you think about how to help make this idea become a reality, you re-alize that you'll need to use multiple tactics. First, you'll need political support to approve such a project, and financial and perhaps instrumental support to pay for building the trail. Here's where your policy tactics come in handy. You build a strong, evidence-based case for the importance of physical activity to community residents and you present it to local leaders. You explain that the idea for this program emerged from the residents themselves and is supported by a wide range of community organizations, agencies, and coalitions. You make it clear that if the local leaders support the plan, they can rightfully claim credit for it in the next election. To strengthen your influence on deci-sion makers, you also take your case directly to the public. That's when your media advocacy tactics come into play. You set a clear advocacy objective—to gain public and political support for building a walking trail in the com-munity. You identify your key audience members—decision makers in the mayor's office and city council, plus the general public. You keep your message simple and clear—if we want to be a healthy community, we must provide our citizens with the opportunity to be healthy. You present a solu-tion—we must build a walking trail.

When approval for the idea is granted, you work closely with other pro-gram partners to make it happen. Here's another way in which community participation pays off. The owner of the home supply store offers to lend a wood chipper to help create mulch for the surface of the walking trail. The Heart Health Coalition volunteers its members' services on weekends to help measure and clear a path for the trail. A local home builder donates leftover concrete to help secure milepost markers around the trail. And so the trail gets built.

Many health promotion practitioners would stop here. But you realize that building the trail alone will not be enough to achieve the broader pro-gram objectives of decreasing sedentary lifestyle and improving quality of life. People in the community need to be made aware of the trail and sold on its virtues. Here, your health communication tactics can help. Finally, you want people to use the trail on a regular basis, thereby establishing a behavioral routine of exercise. So you ensure that the trail includes a system to monitor each individual's exercise frequency, intensity, and duration and provide participants with tailored feedback to reinforce their progress. How do you accomplish this? You install a magnetic card reader at the trailhead and issue walking-trail cards to all community residents who use the trail. You teach them to wear their cards when they visit the trail. Then, each time they pass the card reader, it records their time and distance. A computer translates these data into individualized weekly reports and mails them to each trail user.

In creating this program, you have used policy and media advocacy tactics (securing the support of local decision makers and the general public), community participation and environmental intervention tactics (building the trail itself), health communication tactics (to promote awareness and use of the trail), and tailored communication (to promote and reinforce behavior change).

SUMMARY

The word "create" means to cause or bring about, to produce, and to originate. The creative energy of most practitioners really starts to flow when they reach the point of framing the approach and detailing the tactics that will make up their health promotion program. How do we get that "just right" approach to media advocacy, an innovative policy initiative, or the unique message that reaches people and promotes action heretofore ignored?

While such innovative actions could result from a stroke of creative genius, they are much more likely to be the product of a less dramatic process. Their origin might be the creation of a simpler message, elaboration of a current method, or temporary shift of the emphasis away from health and toward a social or economic concern. In this chapter, the key message is that the creative process will have a greater chance of leading to effective health promotion tactics if all of the prior steps of the planning process are in alignment.

When things get difficult (and they will) and your program won't work the way you had hoped (and it may not), identify and remember those mistakes long enough to avoid repeating them! Our capacity to learn from false starts is one of the most important and practical steps toward innovation.

ENDNOTES

1. Reid DJ, Killoran AJ, McNeill AD, Chambers JS. Choosing the most effective health promotion option for reducing a nation's smoking prevalence. *Tobacco Control.* 1992;1:185–197. This article offers a very easy-to-follow and practical illustration of how to envision many different methods being applied comprehensively to a single, priority health problem. In the case story, Colonel Gayle's "modified" version of the Reid et al. matrix was easy to create, given the thoughtful detail put into the original.

2. For a clear description of how objectives are critical building blocks for developing effective interventions, we recommend Puska P, Yuomilehto J, Nissinen A, Vartiainen E. *The North Karelia Project 20-year Results and Experiences.* Helsinki, Finland: National Public Health Institute and WHO Europe; 1995; 44–47.

3. Brownson RC, Koffman DM, Novotny T, Hughes RG, Eriksen MP. Environmental and policy interventions to control tobacco use and prevent cardiovascular disease. *Health Educ Q.* 1995;22(4):478–498.

4. The resources we used to create this section on health communications are the same resources we turn to in our own planning and research activity: *Making Health Communications Work: A Planner's Guide.* Washington, DC: U.S. Department of Health and Human Services, NIH publication No. 89-1493, 1989; *Communication: A Guide for Managers of National Diarrheal Disease Control Programmes.* Geneva: World Health Organization, Diarrheal Control Programme; 1987; *The CDC Health Communication Book: A Primer on Risk Communication Principles and Practices.* Atlanta: Agency for Toxic Substances and Disease Registry, U.S. Department of Health and Human Services; 1994; and Manoff RK. *Social Marketing: New Imperative for Public Health.* New York: Prager Publishers; 1985.

5. We have chosen to use a "questions" rather than a "steps" format in this context because the latter often implies a linear, prescribed sequence of actions. The critical analysis phase of health communication is primarily an interactive process, where insights gained on one issue will trigger revisiting a prior question. To that extent, the priority should not be the order in which questions are asked, just that they are asked in the first place.

6. Some messages may appear to be more compelling, and thus better attended to, than others—for example, "Dangerous Curve, Slow to 15 m.p.h." Even a message like that could go unattended if it were in a language different from that of the receiver, or were too small or inadequately lit to be read.

7. Figure 6.2 was taken from *Communication: A Guide for Managers of National Diarrheal Disease Control Programmes.* Geneva: World Health Organization; 1987:30.

8. Maibach E, Parrott RL, eds. *Designing Health Messages.* Thousand Oaks, CA: Sage Publications; 1995.

9. Lefebvre CR, Doner L, Johnston C, Loughrey K, Balch GI, Sutton SM. Use of database marketing and consumer-based health communication in message design. In: Maibach E, Parrott RL, eds. *Designing Health Messages.* Thousand Oaks, CA: Sage Publications; 1995.

10. The "5 a Day" program was initiated in 1988 by the California State Department of Health Service under a grant from the National Cancer Institute (NCI). The purpose of the program was to promote increases in fruit and vegetable consumption. Based upon the success of the California experience, "5 a Day" became a national campaign in 1991 with the support of the NCI.

11. A full report of the methods and finding of this evaluation can be found in Kreuter Marshall W, Kreuter Matthew W, Hearn M. *A National Assessment of Reach to Recovery.* Atlanta: American Cancer Society; 1992. The specific reference to the notion of sender credibility is found on page 28 of the report.

12. Green LW, Kreuter MW. *Health Promotion Planning: An Educational and Environmental Approach.* Menlo Park, CA: Mayfield Publishing; 1990:4–5.

13. Chapman S, Lupton D. *The Fight for Public Health: Principles and Practice of Media Advocacy.* London: BMJ Publishing; 1994:135.
14. McKinlay J. A case for refocusing upstream: the political economy of illness. In: Conrad R, Kerns R, eds. *The Sociology of Health and Illness.* New York: St. Martin's Press; 1986:484–498.
15. For example, see Wallack L. Mass communication and health promotion: a critical perspective. In: Rice R, Atkin C, eds. *Public Communication Campaigns.* Newbury Park, CA: Sage Publications; 1990; Wallack L, Dorfman L, Jernigan D, Themba M. *Media Advocacy and Public Health: Power for Prevention.* Newbury Park, CA: Sage Publications; 1993; Wallack L, Dorfman L. Television news, hegemony, and health. *Am J Public Health.* 1992;82:125; and Chapman S, Lupton D. *The Fight for Public Health: Principles and Practice of Media Advocacy.* London: BMJ Publishing; 1994.
16. Larry Wallack and Lori Dorfman, through the Berkeley Media Studies Group, conduct workshops and training on various aspects of media advocacy. Their work has been featured nationally in many settings, including the Promoting Public Health in an Era of Change training programs sponsored by the User Liaison Program of the Agency for Health Care, the Kansas Health Foundation's annual Health Leadership Institute, and World Conference Mental Health in Atlanta, 2001.
17. For more details on the notion of piggybacking, see Ryan C. *Prime Time Activism.* Boston: South End Press; 1991; and Wallack L, Dorfman L, Jernigan D, Themba M. *Media Advocacy and Public Health: Power for Prevention.* Newbury Park, CA: Sage Publications; 1993;93.
18. The-wei H, Hai-yen S, Keeler T. Reducing cigarette consumption in California: tobacco taxes versus an anti-smoking media campaign. *Am J Public Health.* 1995;85:1218–1222.
19. Average Annual Number of Deaths, 1995–1999, Centers for Disease Control and Prevention. *Morbidity and Mortality Weekly Reports.* 2002;51(14):300–303.
20. Simmons S. New cig is aimed at black smokers: Uptown to be tested here. *Philadelphia Daily News.* December 14, 1989, p. 51.
21. Dagnoli J. RJR's Uptown targets blacks. *Advertising Age.* December 18, 1989.
22. Sutton CD. The coalition against Uptown cigarettes: marketing practices and community mobilization November 21, 1993 (www.onyx-group.com/Uptown1.htm).
23. Cotton P. Tobacco foes attack ads that target women, minorities, teens and the poor. *JAMA.* 1990;264(12):1505.
24. See King AC, Jeffrey RW, Fidinger F. Environmental and policy approaches to cardiovascular disease prevention though physical activity: issues and opportunities. *Health Education Q.* 1995;22:499–511; Sallis JF, Bauman A, Pratt M. Environmental and policy interventions to promote physical activity. *Am J Preventive Medicine.* 1998;15(4):379–397; and Schmid TL, Pratt M, Howze E. Policy as intervention: environmental and policy approaches to the prevention of cardiovascular disease. *Am J Public Health.* 1995;85:1207–1211.
25. Prochaska JO, DiClemente CC. In search of how people change: applications to addictive behaviors. *Am Psychologist.* 1992;47(9):1102–1114; Becker MH, ed. The health belief model and personal health behavior. *Health Education Monographs.* 1974;2:324–473; and Bandura A. Toward a unifying theory of behavior change. *Psychological Review.* 1977;84(2):191–215.

26. Strecher VJ, Kreuter MW, Den Boer DJ, Korbrin S, Hospers HJ, Skinner CS. The effects of computer-tailored smoking cessation messages in family practice settings. *J Fam Prac.* 1994;39(3):262–270.
27. Rimer BK, Orleans CT, Fleisher L, Cristinzo S, Resch N, Telepchak J, et al. Does tailoring matter? The impact of a tailored guide on ratings and short-term smoking-related outcomes for older smokers. *Health Education Research.* 1994; 9(1):69–84.
28. Campbell MK, DeVellis BM, Strecher VJ, Ammerman AS, DeVellis RF, Sandler RS. The impact of message tailoring on dietary behavior change for disease prevention in primary care settings. *Am J Public Health.* 1994;84(5):783–787.
29. Skinner CS, Strecher VJ, Hospers H. Physician recommendations for mammography: do tailored messages make a difference? *Am J Public Health.* 1994: 84(1):43–49.
30. The process of developing tailored messages requires the planner (or team of planners) to have ready access to the following competencies: (1) educational and behavioral theory, (2) data collection (questionnaire design) based on theory, (3) data analysis, (4) creation of multiple messages and testing of those messages, and (5) creation of the algorithms that will link selected communications and behavioral characteristics with the appropriate message from a library of health messages.
31. It is not our intention to go into detail about the computer programming aspects of tailoring. However, as computer technology in public health continues to expand, practitioners will find it useful to have some conceptual understanding of the process.

Step 4 is to develop a database. Once the tailoring assessment has been administered, participants' responses must be recorded in a way that allows them to be easily converted into the appropriate tailored messages. Creating a computer database with at least one data field for each assessment question is the simplest way to accomplish this. Each question in the assessment tool must be assigned a variable name. For example, a question assessing barriers to quitting smoking (such as "What would keep you from quitting smoking?") might be named Q.SMK.BARRIER, shorthand for "question about smoking cessation barriers." There might be four response options for this question: fear of failing, stress, concern about weight gain, and peer pressure; they would be numbered 1, 2, 3, and 4, respectively. Thus, if Jane Doe's record in the database showed a value of 3 in the field named Q.SMK.BARRIER, we would conclude that she said that concern about weight gain might keep her from quitting smoking.

In Step 5, the main task is to fit the names of our variables to each tailored message. In the previous step, the barrier for the smoker who was concerned about gaining weight might be called TM.SMK.BAR.WEIGHT, shorthand for "tailored message about smoking cessation barrier weight gain." When all tailored messages have been named, they should be placed together in a single document. This document forms the tailored-message library.

Tailoring algorithms are formed by using "if/then" logic statements to join each question variable with its related tailored messages. In our present example, putting these two together gives us an algorithm that might read "if Q.SMK.BARRIER = 3 then put TM.SMK.BAR.WEIGHT in the tailored quit smoking plan." In other words, if Jane Doe said concern about weight gain would keep her from quitting, give her the tailored message addressing weight gain as a barrier to cessation.

At its simplest level, tailoring printed materials is nothing more than a complex print-merge function in most word-processing programs. When you send a form letter to 100 different persons using print merge, the letter contains open spaces, or fields, for the first name, last name, street address, city, state, and ZIP code. When this letter is merged with a data file containing the names and addresses of the 100 persons, it produces 100 personalized letters. In tailoring, instead of having a small field at the top of the letter allocated to the variable "first name," you might have a field consuming one-third of the page that is allocated to a message about barriers to quitting smoking. When the tailoring algorithms are merged with an individual's responses from the database, the appropriate quit-smoking-barrier message is pulled from the tailored-message library and placed into the participant's feedback.

When all tailoring algorithms have been created, they must be tested extensively. Providing the wrong message to a person (a "tailoring misfire") will not only compromise the credibility of the program, but could also harm the message recipient if inappropriate actions are recommended.

32. Prochaska JO, DiClemente CC, Norcross JC. In search of how people change: applications to addictive behaviors. *Am Psychologist.* 1992;47:1102–1114.
33. Bandura A. *Social Foundations of Thought and Action.* Englewood Cliffs, NJ: Prentice-Hall; 1986.

CHAPTER 7

Steering Versus Rowing

Case Story
JAMESON

Remember the first case story about Linda Thomas? Well, Linda Thomas was not the only one who responded to Fran Martin's remarks about "why we do what we do." Dr. Gordon Jameson—the director of the Tri-County Health Department (TCHD) and Linda Thomas's boss—was also in the audience. Although his given name was Gordon, everyone outside of his professional life called him Jameson—even his mother and father! When he was a young boy, he asked his parents why they didn't call him by his given name. They told him that one month after he was born, a very bad man had tried to swindle them out of some property that had been in the family for decades. They explained that the nasty encounter left a lot of bad feelings behind—and the man's name was Gordon. From that point on, he was Jameson.

Dr. Martin's remarks had made Jameson recall his magnetic pull to public health two decades before. In addition to being a family practice physician, he had served in the Peace Corps in Ghana. It was his experience in Ghana that convinced him that he could do more good by preventing than by repairing. He had his own handwritten modification to the Hippocratic oath hanging on his office wall: "Do good—do your best to do no harm, and before you do either, ask people if they really want your help in the first place!" He suspected that he shared this "Peace Corps gene" with many of his colleagues.

Jameson wondered, though, if his staff shared these motivations. In fact, he had been troubled throughout Dr. Martin's lecture by a sense that in his own health department, the ideals of public health were not translated into a daily sense of mission and accomplishment. Indeed, he felt a distinct lack of enthusiasm about leaving the glow of her inspiring remarks and returning to the daily grind of the TCHD: insufficient resources, staff grievances, media scrutiny, and all the other difficulties that seemed to take up more and more of each day.

Jameson waited patiently as Dr. Martin fielded the usual flurry of inquiries that follow a provocative and stimulating presentation. As a reward for being the last person in line, Jameson suddenly found that he had her undivided attention. He introduced himself, then told Dr. Martin how much he

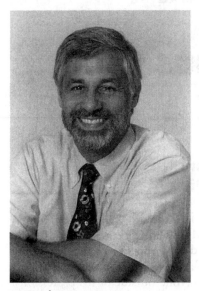

Dr. Gordon Jameson

had appreciated her words and how he wished more of his staff could have attended the lecture. As their conversation continued, he found himself wondering out loud about whether his staff shared his own views of public health, and whether they, too, felt overwhelmed by the daily struggles their work entailed.

Dr. Martin reassured him that his concerns were far from unique. However, she was not going to let him off the hook so easily.

"What are you planning to do about it?" she demanded. Jameson was somewhat taken aback. He had expected to do some more leisurely thinking (and perhaps commiserating!) before swinging into action. Besides, he had arranged a management retreat for the staff a few months ago. Somewhat sheepishly, he offered this information to Dr. Martin as evidence of his efforts.

"A retreat!" she said, in mock horror.

"Well," stammered Jameson, trying hard to recover, and knowing full well that the retreat had fallen short of his expectations, "Well, I'm open to suggestions!" In the back of his mind, an appealing vision was taking shape — a vision of Dr. Martin swooping into the TCHD and motivating the troops.

But swooping was not on Dr. Martin's agenda. "You and your staff have to work on this problem yourselves," she said, somewhat sternly. "And not during a retreat!" Correctly interpreting the misgivings in his expression, she relented. "I do know some people who could help you get started, though, if you'd like."

Dr. Martin jotted down three names on the back of her business card. She circled the middle name and said, "All three of these people are first rate, but this one would be my first choice. He's very insightful, and he's been in the trenches. Best of all, he lives in Atlanta, only 100 miles from your health department—and he loves to drive!" Relieved at having a concrete task ahead of him, Jameson thanked Dr. Martin for her remarks and suggestions and agreed to call one of the consultants.

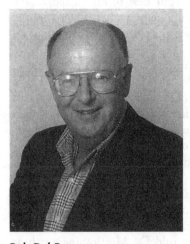

Bob Del Rey

On the first try, Jameson made telephone contact with Bob Del Rey, the man in the middle of Fran Martin's list. Surely, he thought, this was a good sign! When Bob picked up the phone, Jameson was instantly reminded of his own teenage years when he heard—could it be?—ZZ Top blaring in the background. Bob sounded a little out of breath. "Just a minute!" he said, a little louder than necessary. "I'll turn that down!"

When Bob returned to the phone, Jameson explained who he was and how he had ended up calling. They chatted for a few moments about how terrific Fran Martin was, and then Bob asked what his caller had in mind.

Jameson briefly described the size and scope of the health department, and outlined his managerial concerns. Bob asked Jameson to send him some details about the health department's organization, any recent planning documents, and a brief recap of his main concerns. In exchange, Jameson asked Bob to send his résumé. At the end of the conversation, they were on a first-name basis—or, in Jameson's case, close enough!

The two men agreed to talk on the phone again after Bob had a chance to review the materials; then Bob would spend two days at the TCHD. He proposed having an initial morning meeting with Jameson alone; in the afternoon and on the following day, he would have one-on-one sessions with the supervisors of all the major departments and a sample of staff throughout the organization. Jameson agreed to make those arrangements.

Meanwhile, Jameson—not doubting Fran Martin's judgment, but intrigued—did some checking on his own. He had a few sources at the CDC, several of whom knew quite a bit about Bob Del Rey. Fortunately, what they had to say was right in line with Dr. Martin's assessment and the information in Bob's résumé.

A graduate of a small liberal-arts college in Iowa, Bob had started out with a commitment to become a dentist. Once his friends questioned whether he really wanted to spend a lifetime groping around in other people's open mouths, however, he turned his interest to a more mundane field: biology. Bob graduated on time in 1964 and immediately joined the U.S. Public Health Service, motivated in part by a strong interest in avoiding the war in Vietnam. His first job, as a venereal disease (VD) investigator tracking down syphilis cases in New York City, made Bob question his decision to abandon dentistry.

At the time, he had no idea that he would retire 30 years later as one of the most effective managers ever to serve the CDC. During his three decades of service, Bob accumulated numerous awards and plaques acknowledging his contributions and achievements, none of which ever made it out of the boxes they came in. The only award he displayed was his first-place team trophy for bowling in 1981.

Jameson looked out of his office window just as a red Porsche pulled into the parking lot—right on time for the meeting they had discussed earlier. The consulting business must be a lucrative one for Bob Del Rey, Jameson thought, although certainly the rates he had quoted seemed very

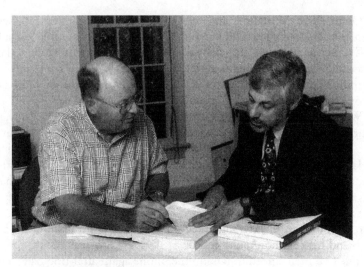

Bob Del Rey and Dr. Gordon Jameson

reasonable. Watching curiously and intently, he was surprised to see a man step out of the car, dressed very comfortably in a short-sleeved shirt, loose-fitting khakis, and decidedly nondesigner tennis shoes. He pulled a battered briefcase from the back seat and strode purposefully into the building. Sure enough, the same figure was soon knocking on Jameson's open door.

After he had greeted Jameson with an introductory "Nice to meet you, Gordon," Bob was treated to the story about the swindler. Bob chuckled, "That's a new one!"

After they had seated themselves, Bob hauled a yellow notepad out of his briefcase and readied himself to take a few notes. "In the material you sent," Bob said, "you indicated that you had a retreat about six months ago with program managers and came up with vision statements and mission statements for their various programs. Did you also undertake any exercises that resulted in the identification of health priorities in your service area?"

"Actually, yes," Jameson replied. "We asked the directors of four programs—maternal and child health, communicable diseases, nursing, and adult health—to give us annual summaries of the encounters they had by disease or reported health problem. Those matched up pretty well with health objectives outlined in the our state's *Healthy People: Health Objectives* document."

"Let me ask you a resource question," Bob continued. "In terms of your total TCHD budget, what portions come from local revenues versus state and federal monies?"

Jameson thought for a second and said, "I don't have the exact numbers off the top of my head, but I can give you a pretty accurate estimate. Approximately 40 percent comes from county and municipal revenues. A little over 35 percent comes from state and federal grants and contracts, most of which reaches us through the state health department. We get another

15 percent in fees from services we provide — our well-baby clinics and immunization programs, for example. A small portion falls into the noncategorical area we call other."

"How about the expenditure side?" Bob asked. "Where does the money go?"

"That's easy," Jameson said, recalling his frequent testimony to the county commissioners. "Nearly 70 percent goes to salaries, well over 25 percent goes to operating costs, only 1.5 percent goes for capital outlay, and the rest is noncategorical."

Bob nodded. He had known in advance what Jameson's answer would be. Now he changed direction. "Okay, of the management challenges you're trying to address, does any one issue or problem stand out in your mind?"

Jameson's eyes searched the floor for a moment. "I couldn't put my finger on any one issue per se. It's just that we always seem to be reacting rather than initiating! Every TCHD employee has a yearly work plan, but I'd bet that more than 50 percent of what we actually do is in response to new initiatives or new problems that come up during the year, few of which are in the work plans."

Bob nodded and smiled knowingly. "Other duties as assigned, eh?"

Jameson thought to himself, "I like this guy."

They completed their discussions over lunch. Jameson handed Bob a schedule of meetings with other staff, as Bob had requested. They agreed that, after Bob completed his interviews, he would return to Atlanta, prepare a summary report with recommendations, and have that report back to Jameson within two weeks.

Bob had prepared a series of questions and planned to ask each person the same questions, regardless of his or her department or rank:

- What is the health department's mission?
- What is your division's mission?
- What role do you play in the health department? In your division?
- How long have you been here?
- How are decisions made here?
- What is a typical day like?
- What helps you do your job?
- What hinders you in doing your job?
- What are the main challenges that the health department faces in the next few years?
- How do others, especially those with a stake in health, view the health department and its role?

In addition, as the opportunity presented itself, Bob asked each employee to loosely track how he or she spent every day for a week — an hour-by-hour summary that showed planned and impromptu meetings, new and old crises, paperwork, supervisory commitments, training, and so forth.

Bob Del Rey was easy to talk to. He expressed a sincere interest in people, but was never overbearing. He had the uncanny ability to be frank and kind at the same time. As he listened, he searched for themes and patterns in the responses people gave to his questions. Bob noted that some of those themes echoed the concerns that Jameson had raised during their one-on-one interview. For example, like Jameson, many of the staff felt frustrated by the back-to-back crises that seemed to be hitting them with increasing frequency. Bob also found that some personnel were unclear about what the health department's highest priorities should be—even some who had attended the retreat together to craft a mission statement. Indeed, several of the interviewees were unaware that a new mission statement even existed.

In their comments about the future, staff were concerned about funding cuts and their effects both on their individual jobs and salaries and on the health department and its ability to provide needed services. Many felt that they were already as lean as they could be, and that the next step would be to turn people away or cut back their hours. Staff uniformly acknowledged Jameson's sincere dedication to his job, and several sympathized with the administrative challenges he faced. As one senior staff member put it, "Who would want his job?"

The staff who saw patients through the department's various clinics also worried that managed-care organizations would underestimate the difficulty of working with the populations that the health department had served for many years. These individuals expressed concerns about whether immunizations, HIV counseling and testing, and other needed services would continue to be provided at the same levels.

Many staff felt that time and resources were not generally available for attending training or educational sessions, nor did they feel well informed about which issues other departments were tackling. Some described the frustration they felt when they had trouble explaining what they did to friends or neighbors, especially with the added stigma of working "for the government." When Bob asked the interviewees how others with a stake in health viewed the health department and its role, the responses were vague. Few staff could identify key stakeholders beyond the Board of Health.

Bob was not surprised by the many complaints he heard from staff about the bureaucratic aspects of their jobs—having to fill out forms showing the same data in different ways, writing endless reports for various state and federal agencies, and rarely seeing a return on these efforts. Some suggested that the bureaucracy and funding streams made them inefficient, and that perhaps the health department should be run more like a business. Surely their counterparts in the private sector didn't have to put up with the combination of uncertainty, scrutiny, and disdain that they did!

Bob's conversations with the staff ended on a positive note when they talked about the chains of events—some planned, some completely random—that had led them to this field. Despite these frustrations, Bob felt that the staff represented a great deal of talent and enthusiasm for public health, and generally respected one another. This was the good news to relay back to the staff and to Jameson.

Bob Del Rey's report back to Jameson was entitled "Opportunities and Challenges for the TCHD." The introductory section included a brief synthesis of the background information on the TCHD that Jameson had turned over to Bob for review. It was followed by a section called "Emerging Issues." Bob had used health status data from the TCHD service area and matched it up with similar indicators for the state of Georgia and for the southeastern region of the United States to make some projections of the health issues most likely to emerge in the TCHD's service area.

The remainder of the report was divided into four components, each of which had been shaped by the information and themes Bob derived from the interviews:

- Essential Services
- Strategic Planning
- Benchmarking
- Private- and Public-Sector Enterprises

For each component, Bob defined the category, explained how staff comments directly or indirectly gave rise to that category, and offered recommendations for action.

In his cover letter to Jameson, Bob included a quote by Max dePree: "The first responsibility of a leader is defining reality."[1]

Bob went on to write:

> In every management situation I can recall over the past 30 years, no single attribute was more critical to building organizational confidence than when the manager or leader was forthcoming with accurate and insightful information about the realities facing the organization. Doubt and mistrust are less likely when leaders seek out and reveal the honest realities of their circumstances, warts included!

Case Analysis

The management "how-to" shelves at bookstores and libraries continue to expand with books on every imaginable managerial challenge. Each book, in turn, adds to the jargon of management. Terms such as total quality management (TQM), quality circles (QCs), learning organizations, reengineering, and many others have seeped into our everyday language.

Unfortunately, no book—including this one—can create good management overnight. Instead, our goal in this section is to examine several basic tenets of good management practice and to ask practitioners to "walk a mile" in the shoes of the supervisor or manager; we have found that practitioners who understand the managerial perspective are more likely than those without such understanding to inform and, in some cases, influence the decisions of their managers and leaders.

We believe that sound management practice is often overlooked, particularly in crisis-driven environments like the TCHD. This omission occurs for a number of reasons. First, people often assume that managerial skill is a "freebie" that the organization gets with any talented, accomplished person. Unfortunately, skill in one area does not always translate into the managerial realm.

Moreover, training and guidance for managerial functions are often nonexistent or perfunctory—such as a one-day workshop on how to supervise employees or work with a difficult colleague. Another set of assumptions represents the opposite problem—a sort of fatalism about individual styles and personalities and their intractable nature. The fact is that "control freaks" and freewheeling artistic types can all be equally good managers, but they may arrive at that point differently.

The management information presented here is divided into two main categories: organizational and individual. An organization is a collection of individuals who must work together to accomplish common goals. The organization and its leadership have some specific elements to contribute to the organization's success, but so do the individuals who make up the organization. Good management is a collective responsibility of every member of the organization. In this case, for instance, both Linda Thomas and Dr. Jameson have specific contributions to make to the successful management of the TCHD. In other words, even if you are not a manager per se, the management skills outlined here should prove useful to you.

MANAGEMENT AND ORGANIZATIONS

Dr. Jameson had already told Bob Del Rey about some of the steps he had taken to define organizational goals. These efforts included the retreat with the department managers, the match between client encounters and published national and state health objectives, and the attempt to create a new mission statement. Unfortunately, as Bob's interviews with staff revealed, these efforts had not built consensus throughout the organization. Recall that some people were unaware of the new mission statement, and others disagreed about what the organization's priorities were.

In this section, we will review the following tools and concepts, which were the framework for Bob Del Rey's report:

- Essential services of public health
- Strategic planning
- Benchmarking
- Private- and public-sector enterprises

Essential Services

One tool that Dr. Jameson and his staff have not yet used to address these types of discrepancies is the essential-services language that we reviewed in Chapter 1. Like the core functions that preceded them, the essential services provide a framework and vocabulary for discussing public health activities. Most organizations will not undertake the entire spectrum of essential services. For example, state and local health departments have different emphases on surveillance (typically heavier at the state level) and personal care services (typically more prevalent at the local level). Community-based organizations, foundations, advocacy groups, hospitals, and others active in public health may each focus on a specific service. In any case, essential-services language offers a way to describe where an organization currently stands and where it might shift its attention in response to its own momentum or the effects of outside forces.

At the TCHD, the essential services could serve as a starting point for discussions about what the TCHD is currently doing and how its activities might change in the future. For example, if (as some staff mentioned) managed-care organizations take over some of the services that are currently provided by staff at the TCHD, what will their roles be? The possibilities include collaborating with managed-care organizations (e.g., by providing outreach services), providing training to staff who are new to population-based services, or even shifting to other services.

Strategic Planning

Anticipating and preparing for the future is an important leadership function for Dr. Jameson and his staff. The process of managing the constant change that affects almost any organization is captured by the strategic planning process.[2] *Strategic planning* is a term that is often misused to refer to a specific document—such as the strategic plan that Dr. Jameson sent to Bob Del Rey. A strategic plan document is one product of a strategic planning process, but it is by no means the only product, nor is it even the most important one. Many organizations struggle through the long meetings and semantic revisions that lead to a strategic plan, then breathe a sigh of relief because they believe that they are finished. In fact, the resulting document is merely a fuzzy snapshot of the organization at a certain point in time, and one that can and should be updated regularly to refine the picture and ensure that it remains accurate. Think of the strategic plan itself as a recording or imprint of a dynamic process—something that participants can refer to over time to refresh their memories, check their assumptions, and measure their progress.

Strategic planning can be undertaken in various ways, at various levels of detail. In fact, it may not even be called strategic planning. Regardless of the name it goes by, the strategic planning process tries to answer three key questions:

1. Where are we now?
2. Where do we want to be?
3. How do we get there?

Each of these issues can have numerous dimensions, such as funding levels, staff skill sets, new products or programs, customer service, collaborative relationships, and so on. The answers will depend, of course, on the contours of each organization and its subunits. For example, at TCHD, it might be useful for each department to examine these questions, and then to come together as a group to see where overlap or divergence exists. Table 7.1 lists common categories addressed through a strategic planning process.

Where Are We Now?

This question leads to a baseline measure of where an organization stands. It typically includes an environmental scan—a sort of "lay of the land," internally and externally. An internal assessment takes a clear, unflinching look at the organization's strengths and weaknesses. An external assessment looks at opportunities and threats, which may sometimes be two sides of the same coin. For example, many public health practitioners view the advent of managed-care organizations as both an opportunity and a threat.

Another tool to help determine where an organization stands is a stakeholder analysis. Who are the key stakeholders for your organization? What do they think of your performance? What criteria do they use to judge your performance?

Where Do We Want to Be?

Future goals should incorporate both short- and long-term time frames—for example, one year as well as four to five years and even a decade into the future. A useful exercise in discussing this question is to have staff think about the future without real-world constraints. Remember Dr. Jameson's "Peace Corps gene"; even goals that sound hopelessly naive or unrealistic may trigger a useful or just plain inspiring discussion. Perhaps some of those real-world barriers to accomplishing lofty goals are not as imposing or immovable as they seemed. Many good ideas and programs got their start with the words, "If only we could . . ."

TABLE 7.1   Ten Strategic Planning Steps

Step 1: Initiate and Agree on a Strategic Planning Process

- Identify key decision makers
- Determine who should be involved (people, units, agencies)

Step 2: Clarify Organizational Mandates

- List mandates ("musts") and sources (charters, policies, rules)
- Determine implications of mandates for current operations
- Determine whether mandates should be changed

Step 3a: Identify and Understand Stakeholders

- Identify internal and external stakeholders
- Determine criteria they use to judge performance
- Determine how they would rate the agency's performance

Step 3b: Develop/Refine Mission Statement and Values

- Clarify purpose of organization; why you do what you do
- Response to key stakeholders
- Philosophy/core values
- Distinct/unique contributions
- Current values; additional values to guide conduct in the future

Step 4: Assess the Environment

- List *internal* strengths and weaknesses
- List *external* opportunities and threats
- Identify options for building on strengths and opportunities, and minimizing weaknesses and threats

Step 5: Identify/Frame Strategic Issues

- Identify challenges to the organization that require immediate action, action in the near future, or monitoring
- Identify consequences of not addressing each issue

Step 6: Formulate Strategies to Manage Issues

- Determine strategies, barriers, and specific actions to address strategic issues
- Develop a first-draft strategic plan listing specific strategies and actions

Step 7: Review and Adopt the Strategic Plan

- Include key internal and external stakeholders

Step 8: Establish an Effective Organizational Vision for the Future

- Describe the "vision of success" for the organization, based on the mission statement, values, and strategies

Step 9: Develop an Effective Implementation Process

- List existing programs and services
- Set priorities
- Determine actions, results, milestones
- Decide who is responsible
- Assign dates/resources

Step 10: Reassess the Strategic Planning Process

- Identify strengths and weaknesses of existing strategies
- Suggest modifications
- Decide which should be maintained, revised, or terminated

How Do We Get There?

Unlike the second question, this one does need to be firmly rooted in reality. What resources are required: money, people, skills, training? What alternative routes exist, if some or all of these resources are unavailable or are not available in the quantities needed? What kinds of new or reinforced collaboration may be required? And the most important questions: Who will be responsible for it, and by when? These responses form the most important part of the written document. It is acceptable to miss these deadlines, but it is also acceptable to expect an explanation—and a modification for the next round of goals and timelines. If timelines and responsibilities are agreed upon and nothing else ever happens, your next planning effort will have to surmount a lot of skepticism, as well it should.

Benchmarking

You have probably noticed that the answers to each of the preceding questions depend on some type of objective measures of what the current situation is and how it changes over time. The national *Healthy People* objectives for the nation are one such measure. As Dr. Jameson pointed out, these goals have been adapted by many states for their own specific circumstances. The benchmarks process described in Chapter 2 is an excellent example of how measurable goals are used to drive activities not only in public health but throughout state government. If Bob Del Rey had asked his TCHD counterparts in Oregon about their organization's goals, chances are they would have been able to provide a succinct list for each department.

Private- and Public-Sector Enterprises

The TCHD staff members interviewed by Bob Del Rey talked about two common aspects of working for a government agency: the frustration of internal bureaucratic procedures and the stigma that outsiders attach to "government work."

More and more politicians find it fashionable to criticize public agencies and public service; they paint pictures of Kafkaesque bureaucratic nightmares featuring anecdotes of wasteful government spending and intrusive regulations. Without engaging in the debate over how much or how little government is enough, suffice it to say that in the realm of public health, government agencies at all levels have quietly and successfully assumed responsibility for a wide variety of health issues that affect us as individuals and as communities.

Public health is a public good—one from which we benefit simultaneously as individuals and as communities. It is certainly in your individual interest that the man standing next to you in line at the bus stop not suffer from tuberculosis. It also happens to be in the interests of the other people in the same line, and of everyone else who may come into casual contact with him throughout the day.

There is no profit incentive to induce a private organization to worry about this possibility. Public health does worry about it, however, and tries to do something about it.

As David Osborne and Ted Gaebler point out in their book, *Reinventing Government,* the differences between government and business enterprises "add up to one conclusion: Government cannot be run like a business."[3] One difference they cite to explain this supposition is the slower pace of government, as decisions must be made more openly and with far more outside scrutiny than those made in business.

Another important distinction is that government cannot choose its customers; by definition, government agencies must serve everyone equally. (In public health, this has historically meant those customers least able to afford and acquire health care services elsewhere—those who are often most resource-intensive.) Flexibility in hiring (and firing) staff is restricted in public agencies.

Finally, as a Ford Foundation official notes in Osborne and Gaebler's book, "In government, all of the incentive is in the direction of not making mistakes. You can have 99 successes and nobody notices, and one mistake and you're dead."

This is not to say that government enterprises can't be improved; certainly they can. In fact, that is the main point of Osborne and Gaebler's book. But no matter how much government enterprises can adapt and benefit from private-sector management techniques and entrepreneurial spirit, the fact remains that fundamental differences persist between the two.

What does this discussion have to do with management? It relates to working with what you have. At the TCHD, some of the problems that staff identified could certainly be improved. These include trying to streamline data collection and reporting (perhaps making better use of automation, if the forms and duplication are not in the TCHD's control). Another topic that staff identified was the view that outsiders have of their work. Certainly a key management task is to keep stakeholders aware of what you are doing, so that the recipients of the information see how they and the community benefit from your actions. Identifying and understanding stockholders— both internal and external—is a critical step in the strategic planning process outlined in Table 7.1. In addition to stakeholder analysis, addressing this shortcoming could involve helping staff communicate with the media and with community members about the services they provide.

Staff should pursue these and other improvements with commitment and energy. However, they must also recognize the constraints of their environment. Indeed, the TCHD cannot be run like a business. As a consequence, some efficiencies and resources are inevitably lost. But this constraint also has a positive aspect, emanating from the organization's mission and contributions to the public's health.

Budgeting

Budgeting is an important management skill, whether the numbers in question relate to a new initiative generated by a strategic plan, a grant request, or an agency's or division's annual operating budget. An accurate, realistic budget signals that a manager has a realistic sense of what is required and is willing to be held accountable for the resources allocated to an initiative or program.

Budgets answer a basic question: What will it cost to do this? To answer this question, always consider your audience and any specific requirements that the audience might impose. A related issue is how the budget will be used—for example, for ballpark estimates, accountability, or project management. A good rule of thumb is to think of yourself as a reader. Does the budget tell you what you want to know? Is it clear and readable?[4]

Most budgets cover several typical categories. Of course, these will vary depending on the purpose, audience, and funder. Common categories include the following:

- *Personnel costs*—salaries, fringe benefits, projected raises (if the budget covers multiple years). Some budgets portray personnel costs as a percentage of a person's time and salary. (Often, these costs are called FTEs, for "Full-Time Equivalents.") For example, an agency's director might oversee a project that takes about 20 percent of his or her time. This fact could be noted as a line item for the costs associated with that person as 20 percent of his or her annual salary and benefits. Note that this category usually includes the personnel who are part of an organization's salaried staff. Other workers—such as consultants, outreach workers, and polling organizations—are typically listed under "other direct costs."

- *Other direct costs*—These may include travel, equipment, supplies, printing, postage, telephone/Internet expenses, stipends, and consultants or special studies (such as surveys and polls).

- *Indirect costs*—the costs that organizations charge to outsiders (and within organizations as well) to reflect the ongoing costs of administration and general overhead. Sometimes general and administrative costs are listed separately. In any case, it is always wise to check both your agency's and your funders' expectations and rules about how indirect costs will be charged.

Even a complex operating budget can usually be summarized in one or two pages, with supporting detail provided separately. Sometimes, a brief narrative describing key budget categories is helpful as well (and sometimes such a narrative is required).

Regardless of the budget's format and length, make sure that you check your math carefully—and then do so again. Spreadsheets are a terrific resource for quick budget manipulation, but they can also wreak havoc if unchecked errors ripple through a large budget.

MANAGEMENT AND INDIVIDUALS

The human element of the workplace can be its most rewarding as well as its most frustrating feature. Our work lives would certainly be dull if we worked alongside professionals who had no idiosyncrasies or variations. On the other hand, some personal and professional characteristics can be annoying or even destructive, both to individual colleagues and to the delicate "social fabric" of teams.

What are individuals' obligations to a well-managed organization? We believe these fall into several categories, which are discussed in the following sections:

- Information flow
- The supervisory relationship
- Professional development
- Professional identity

Information Flow

The flow of information is radically transforming every aspect of daily life, including the workplace. Computers, with their vast storage and processing capabilities, and now the information superhighway have made instant access to information the norm for many.

What does this trend mean for how organizations are managed? One implication is a pressure (and capability) to decentralize decision making, as there is not enough time to pass information up and down a hierarchy. It also means that individuals may become inundated and often overwhelmed with information. The task before them is to wade through piles of papers (and now hundreds of Web sites) to decide which of these many pieces of information are actually relevant.

The flow of information within an organization is a clear juncture of organizational and individual responsibilities. In the TCHD example, Dr. Jameson and his senior staff need to do a better job of communicating their own sense of priorities and mission to "the troops." But the troops themselves also have a role to play. If you find yourself in the same position as Linda Thomas, without much strategic direction for your ideas and enthusiasm, you now have the tools to request more information from others in the organization. In other words, you should ask yourself and others: Why are we doing this? How will it help us accomplish our objectives? Is this a better use of resources than another project? Why or why not?

Another aspect of information flow is almost too trite to mention. In any organization, rumors about individuals and organizations can develop a life of their own, often to the detriment of individual reputations and organizational effectiveness. At the TCHD, uncertainty about the future creates a ripe climate for this kind of negative speculation. While a certain amount of this kind of gossip is inevitable, much can be avoided by making as much information as possible available to the greatest number of people. Obviously, personnel decisions and other matters must be treated confidentially. However, the results of the strategic planning retreat, the mission statement, even a frank discussion of what the future might hold—all can help allay unnecessary fears among staff. Although Bob Del Rey did not feel that morale was anywhere near a crisis stage at TCHD, he did recognize some early warning signs, and he knew the remedy.

The Supervisory Relationship

Solid supervisory skills are the building blocks of good managerial practice, governing the one-on-one interactions as well as the teams that make up an organization. Specific supervisory roles vary depending on the organization, but most include the following responsibilities:

- Planning and organizing the work that needs to be done
- Managing people—hiring, training, informing, supporting, and evaluating them
- Achieving objectives—making sure that plans are efficiently implemented, setting performance standards, and adapting to changing conditions

There is no single path to being a good supervisor; supervisory styles span a wide range of personality types and styles. No matter what the specific responsibilities and individual styles, though, several aspects of good supervision are necessary:

Know your job and your organization.   Familiarity with the organization's mission, procedures, and functions is essential to monitoring resources and guiding employees.

Maintain high standards for your own performance.   Supervisors need to call upon a range of conceptual, communications, and technical skills. Make sure that your contributions are of the highest caliber.

Lead by example.   Model the high standards and professional behavior you expect of your employees, including timeliness, focus, quality control, fairness, and honesty, among many others.

Delegate effectively.   Peter Drucker, the famed management "guru," has said that "the purpose of delegation is to enable the supervisor to concentrate on his or her own job, not to delegate it away." Appropriate delegation frees up thinking and planning time, gives other employees an opportunity to learn new skills, demonstrates trust and confidence, and can improve decision making by bringing in new ideas and perspectives. Routine tasks, technical issues, and tasks with potential for skill building are all good candidates for delegation. However, delegation is not always the answer. Do not delegate sensitive personnel matters, those requiring confidentiality, crises, or activities that someone expects you (specifically) to complete.

Professional Development

To do their jobs well, staff need to improve their own skills. Some of this improvement can happen through individual initiative, but organizations have an obligation to identify these needs and act on them. Even when limited budgets and scheduling difficulties hinder attendance at conferences and other training events, professional development can still occur. Opportunities include bringing outside trainers in to work with a group from a city or region, using satellite or video capabilities to transfer knowledge (followed by an interactive discussion among participants on site), and holding informal brown-bag lunches to share new information or ideas.

Ideally, professional development will be tied to individual performance through the performance review process, during which individual staff members work with their supervisors to identify areas where training would be helpful. A secondary step is to assess training needs across the organization, to see which might be relevant to a group of people or to a particular time in their careers.

Professional Identity

Each of us brings a professional persona to the workplace, composed in part of our personality, our previous work experience, and the influence of a particular discipline or training, among many other factors. Each organization also has expectations of what constitutes professional (and unprofessional) behavior, whether they are articulated or not. In discussing this often-implicit aspect of the workplace, Bob Del Rey often mentioned an example from his wife's work as a kindergarten teacher. As a group, Bob's wife and her colleagues got together to decide what it meant to be a professional kindergarten teacher. Their list was not long—in fact, it easily fit on a page. The pithy statement described what they valued about their professional identity and what they expected of one another in dealing with peers, students, parents, and school administrators. This type of assessment is a useful exercise for any group of people working together, since many of these assumptions may not be equally self-evident to everyone.

SUMMARY

Why do we do what we do? This question opened this book, and we have returned to it in this final chapter. Public health practitioners are fortunate to work in a field that many consider a calling—one that combines compassion for others with elements of activism, innovation, and challenge. However, even the most motivated individuals and the most well-intentioned leaders of organizations can falter when they try to translate their enthusiasm and interests into day-to-day practice.

In this chapter, we have presented some tools for gauging an organization's health, setting priorities, and managing how work gets done. We believe that it is important for everyone in an organization to understand how they contribute to the organization's work. In this sense, solid management is not solely the responsibility of the organization's leaders and senior staff. While managers may do more steering than rowing, it is important for all employees to do a little of both—and to know when each is appropriate.

We hope that each of the chapters in this book has helped you formulate your own answers to Fran Martin's probing question, and that you will apply this insight as you put *Ideas That Work* to work in your community.
Good luck!

ENDNOTES

1. dePree M. *Leadership Is an Art.* New York: Doubleday/Currency; 1989.
2. An excellent strategic planning resource is Bryson J. *Strategic Planning for Public and Nonprofit Organizations.* San Francisco: Jossey-Bass; 1995. The accompanying workbook, *Creating and Implementing Your Strategic Plan,* provides sample worksheets and exercises for conducting a strategic planning process. Another useful resource is Allison M, Kay J. *Strategic Planning for Nonprofit Organizations: A Practical Guide and Workbook.* The Support Center for Nonprofit Management; 1997.
3. Osborne D, Gaebler T. *Reinventing Government: How the Entrepreneurial Spirit Is Transforming the Public Sector.* Reading, MA: Addison-Wesley; 1992.
4. For a useful guide on preparing complex budgets, see the budgeting chapter in Gooch JM. *Writing Winning Proposals.* Council for Advancement and Support of Education; 1986.

Index

Adoption, theory of, 133–138
Alinsky, Saul, 124
Alma-Ata Declaration (1974), 61
Assessment
    defined, 10
    MAPP, 36
Assessment Protocol for Excellence in
    Public Health (APEX/PH), 35
Assurance, defined, 10
Australia, diagnostic approach, 99–104

Bandura, A., 129
Behavioral risk factors, 39
*Behavioral Risk Factors Surveillance System
    (BRFSS)*, 39
Benchmarking, 202
Berry, Wendell, 66–67
Brownson, R. C., 154
Budgeting, 204–205

Centers for Disease Control and Prevention
    (CDC), 38–40, 68
    Framework for Program Evaluation,
        105–108
    National Center for Health Statistics
        (NCHS), 38, 40
Change, targets for
    create a matrix, 93–95
    determine changeability, 90–93
    determine factor importance, 90
    differentiate between behavioral and
        environmental factors, 89
    list risk factors, 88–89
    set objectives, 95
    shorten the list, 89–90
    theory and, 125
Channels, communication, 159–161
Chapman, Simon, 161
Checkmate case story, 147–152
Communication. *See* Health
    communication tactic

Community Benchmarking
    Collaborative, 43
Community Capacity theory,
    138–139, 140
Community Coalition Action theory,
    138–140
Community Health Status Assessment
    (CHSA), 36
Community participation, 35
Community themes and strength
    assessment, 36
Compatibility, 135, 136–137
Complexity, 135, 137
Conclusions, justify, 108
Costs, tactics and, 153–154
Court of Public Opinion case story, 51–59
Creativity, tactics and, 154

Data
    case story, 17–34
    finding, 38–40
    help from other people, 41
    hospital discharge, 38–39
    interpreting, 41–42
    local use of, 43, 47
    mortality, 38
    national, 39–40
    resources and models, 35–36
    steps for collecting and organizing,
        37–38
    used to stimulate action, 42–43
Decisions, takes and making informed, 153
dePree, Max, 197
Designing Health Messages (Maibach and
    Parrott), 159
Diffusion of Innovations theory, 133–138
Dorfman, Lori, 163–165

Enabling factors, 97–98
Environmental actions, as a tactic,
    150–151, 174–177

Evaluation, program, 104–112
Evidence, gather and analyze, 107
    case example, 109–112

Foege, William, 22
Framework for Program Evaluation (CDC),
    105–108
Freire, Paulo, 124
Future of Public Health, The, 10

Gaebler, Ted, 203
Georgia Public Health Association
    (GPHA), 1
Government, resource allocation and role
    of, 17–18
Green, Lawrence, 41, 61–62

Health Belief Model (HBM), 126–128
Health communication tactic, 150–151
    channels, 159–161
    messages, determining, 158–159
    perceived costs, 157–158
    role of, 155–156
    target audience, 156–157
Health Communities, 42
Health Promotion and Chronic Disease
    Prevention (HPCDP), cancer
    prevention proposal
    case analysis, 32–34
    final draft, 32
    first draft, 28–31
    input from epidemiologist,
        25–28
    staff meeting and input, 18–25
Healthy Cities, 42
*Healthy People 2010: National Health
    Promotion and Disease Prevention
    Objectives,* 39, 67
Hospital discharge data, 38–39

Information flow, 205–206

Jackson, Joseph, 33

W.K. Kellogg Foundation, 42

Lessons, ensure use and share learned,
    108–109
Lewin, Kurt, 143
Local Public Health System Assessment
    (LPHSA), 36
Longview Health Department,
    109–112

Macro International, 68
Maibach, E., 159
*Making Health Communications Work: A
    Planner's Guide,* 159
Management and individuals
    information flow, 205–206
    professional development, 207
    professional identity, 207
    supervisory relationship, 206–207
Management and organizations, 198
    benchmarking, 202
    budgeting, 204–205
    essential services, 199
    private- and public-sector enterprises,
        202–203
    strategic planning, 199–202
*Manual of the International Statistical
    Classification of Diseases, Injuries,
    and Causes of Death,* 38
McGinnis, Michael, 22
Measuring for Success 2000, 43
Measuring for Success 2001, 43, 47
Media advocacy, 150–151, 161–162
    anticipation, 166
    framing for access, 165
    framing for content, 166
    newspaper story example, 166–168
    steps, 163–165
Minkler, Meredith, 124
Mission statements, importance of, 9–12
Missouri Health Foundation
    (MHF), 8–9
Mobilizing for Action through Planning
    and Partnerships (MAPP),
    35–38, 42
Mortality data, locating, 38

National Association of County and City
    Health Officials (NACCHO), 42
National Center for Health Statistics
    (NCHS), 38, 40
National data, 39–40
National Institutes of Health, 159
Nisker, Scoop, 163
North Carolina Report Card, 43–47

Objectives to stay focused, tactics and,
    152–153
Observability, 135, 137–138
Old Horse case story, 115–123
Osborne, David, 203
Our Kids Count Coalition, case story,
    79–87

Parrott, R. L., 159
Participation
    case story, 51–59
    defined, 59–60
    importance of, 60–67
    promoting political and public support,
        67–73
    strategies for heightening public
        awareness, 73–75
Participation, problems with
    burnout, 63–64
    competing agendas, 63
    lack of community, 65–66
    misrepresentation by media, 64–65
    outside groups resist your plans,
        62–63
Pertschuk, Mike, 154
Planned Approach to Community Health
    (PATCH), 35, 42
Plans
    assumptions, 88
    diagnostic approach, 99–104
    evaluation, 104–112
    identifying causes, 96–98
    Our Kids Count Coalition, case story,
        79–87
    targets for change, 88–95
Policy and regulatory actions, as a tactic,
    150–151, 168–174
Policy development, defined, 10
Political and public support, promoting,
    67–73
Precede-Proceed model, 88, 96, 126, 131
Predisposing factors, 96–97
Professional development, 207
Professional identity, 207
Program priorities, influence of individuals
    on, 14–15
Public awareness, strategies for heightening,
    73–75
Public health
    defined, 75–76
    functions of, 10
Public health in America, assumptions,
    6–8
Public support, promoting, 67–73
Putnam, Robert, 141

Reasoned Action, theory of, 131–133
Reid, Donald, 150
Reinforcing factors, 97
Reinventing Government (Osborne and
    Gaebler), 203

Relative advantage, 135–136
Robert Wood Johnson Foundation, 42
Rose, Geoffrey, 68
Russell, Bill, 9

Seattle, Washington, *E. coli* outbreak in,
    10–12
Self-Efficacy, 128–131
Simplicity, tactics and, 153
Social Capital theory, 138–139,
    141–143
Stakeholders, engage, 106
*Strategy of Preventive Medicine,
    The* (Rose), 68
Supervisory relationship, 206–207
Sustainable Communities and the Center
    for Civic Partnerships, 42

Tactics
    Checkmate case story, 147–152
    combining, to influence
        problems, 154
    costs and, 153–154
    creativity, use of, 154
    environmental actions, 150–151,
        174–177
    health communication, 150–151,
        155–161
    make informed decisions, 153
    media advocacy, 150–151, 161–168
    objectives to stay focused, 152–153
    policy and regulatory actions, 150–151,
        168–174
    simplicity and, 153
    tailoring, 150–151, 177–184
    use of multiple, 184–186
Tailoring, as a tactic, 150–151, 177–184
Theories
    defined, 123–124
    Community Capacity, 138–139, 140
    Community Coalition Action,
        138–140
    Diffusion of Innovations, 133–138
    Health Belief Model, 126–128
    Old Horse case story, 115–123
    relevancy of, 125–126
    Self-Efficacy, 128–131
    Social Capital, 138–139, 141–143
    targets of change and, 125
    Theory of Reasoned Action, 131–133
Trialability, 135, 137
Tri-County Health Department (TCHD),
    2, 3, 5–6, 8

Turning Point: Collaborating for a new Century in Public Health, 42–43

University of Washington, School of Public Health, 42

Wallack, Larry, 163–165
Wilber, Ken, 41

Willett, Bruce, 18
Winslow, C.E.A., 75–76

Youth Risk Behavior Surveillance System (YRBSS), 39
Youth Tobacco Survey (YTS), 39